Y's Way to
WATER
EXERCISE
INSTRUCTOR'S GUIDE

Joseph A. Krasevec

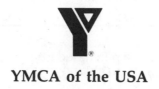

YMCA of the USA

Library of Congress Cataloging-in-Publication Data

Krasevec, Joseph A.
    Y's way to water exercise instructor's guide/Joseph A. Krasevec.
        p. cm.
    Bibliography: p.
    ISBN 0-87322-221-0
    1. Aquatic exercises.   I. National Council of the Young Men's
Christian Associations of the United States of America.   II. Title
RA781.17.K74   1989
613.7'1–dc19   88-30384
                                                                                    CIP

ISBN: 0-87322-221-0

Copyright © 1989 National Council of Young Men's Christian Associations of the United States of America

Published for the YMCA of the USA by Human Kinetics Publishers, Inc.

Cover photo: Kirk Schlea/Berg and Associates.

Printed in the United States of America

10   9   8   7   6   5   4   3   2   1

Copies of this book may be purchased from the YMCA Program Store,
Box 5077, Champaign, IL 61825-5077, (217) 351-5077.

Contents

Preface

The YMCA has long been a proponent of water exercise. In 1982 the YMCA published its first instructional book on water exercise, *Physical Fitness Through Water Exercise*. To respond to the tremendous growth and interest in this activity and to demonstrate its commitment to leadership in the area of physical fitness, the YMCA has produced the Y's Way to Water Exercise program. This program's content is based on HydroRobics, an internationally recognized program developed by Joseph A. Krasevec and Diane Grimes that is consistent with the best programs now being conducted by YMCAs across the country.

The *Y's Way to Water Exercise Instructor's Guide* will help you develop and conduct enjoyable, effective water exercise programs. Chapter 1 provides basic information about the concept of water exercise; unique features about the Y's program; and suggestions on how to use the participant's text, *Y's Way to Water Exercise*, as well as this book. Additional information is presented in chapter 2 on the physical characteristics of water and on research that substantiates the physical benefits of water exercise.

Chapter 3 explains the standard concepts of physical fitness. These training principles are reviewed and applied to water exercise.

Teaching methodology is a vital concern of every fitness instructor. Chapter 4 discusses the primary attributes of a successful instructor, the steps to teaching a new exercise, and a variety of teaching techniques. Sections devoted to motivational strategies and pre- and post-testing are also included.

The YMCA's emphasis on program safety is reflected in chapter 5, which discusses administrative safety planning and class safety. Exercise precautions and danger signs are specified in this chapter. Information on your responsibility as instructor to act prudently and reasonably is highlighted with a list of dos and don'ts of teaching a class safely.

Chapter 6 provides lesson plans for three levels of instruction: beginning, intermediate, and advanced. Also included in the lesson plans are suggested minilectures on a variety of fitness topics.

As many students will be exercising to lose or maintain weight, chapter 7 has pertinent information on nutrition and how food and its component nutrients can affect health and physical appearance.

Positive and negative feedback help many instructors improve their classes. Chapter 8 discusses the need for your students to evaluate both you and the program. Evaluation forms are provided.

A number of appendices are included in this book to provide you with additional examples and helpful information. Appendix A contains minilecture outlines for all three levels of instruction. Appendix B is a complete example of circuit training, and Appendix C describes water games that can add fun to water exercise class. The water jug exercises in Appendix D are helpful if your pool does not have gutters for exercisers to hold on to as they work out. Medical history and screening forms, along with liability forms, appear in Appendix E. The last appendix, Appendix F, is a rating list of the intensity of each aerobic exercise to guide you in customizing exercise routines for your class.

This book, used in conjunction with the *Y's Way to Water Exercise text*, should give you as an aquatics director or instructor all the information you need to implement water exercise programs. Lesson plans and administrative tasks are described in this instructor's guide; descriptions and illustrations of the exercises appear in the participant's text.

Participants should have their own copies of *Y's Way to Water Exercise*. (You may want to include the cost of the book in the program fee.) That book will provide them not only with directions for all exercises but also with additional information about physical fitness. Besides benefiting the individual participant, this can help the success of the class—a person who learns the basic concepts of physical fitness is more likely to approach a fitness program with interest and enthusiasm.

Use of these materials by both you and the participants should make your water exercise class fun and rewarding in the best tradition of the Y.

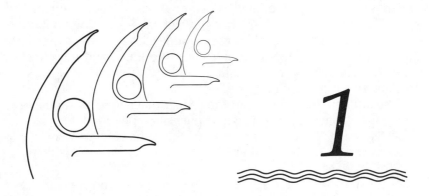

Introduction

Water exercise is coming into its own! It has found a prominent niche among the innumerable fitness activities available to Americans today. With a long tradition, but previously overshadowed by more popular forms of aerobic activities, water exercise classes are increasing in number at a rapid rate.

The Increasing Popularity of Water Exercise

One of the earliest uses of water exercise was as *hydrotherapy*, a form of rehabilitation for specific types of postsurgical cases. Since then water exercise has branched out to serve various purposes and is most popular today as a general form of exercise. The current popularity of water exercise is evidenced by the recent multitude of books written about it and the growing number of water exercise devices that have been developed. Furthermore, recent national polls have indicated that not only are more Americans participating in general exercise, but many are looking to the water for safe, effective physical fitness programs.

Why People Are Attracted to Water Exercise

Many people believe that water exercise has some advantages over exercise in comparable land-based programs. Most important is the water's buoyant effect on the body, which takes the "jolt" out of exercise. Because the immersed portion of one's body is 90 percent lighter in the water, less stress is generated in the joints and muscle tissue, greatly reducing the risk of injury. Added to this is the water's massaging effect, soothing muscles.

The pool environment also represents a place to relax and have fun. Participants often engage in light conversation before, during, and after exercise. Also, like choreographed aerobic exercise classes, most water exercise programs are conducted with music, which reduces the drudgery of exercise.

Some forms of exercise are threatening to those who are embarrassed by their physical awkwardness. Water exercise works for them because the water's buoyancy allows them to be more agile.

As if these weren't enough reasons to be attracted to water exercise, participants don't even need to know how to swim: The exercises are performed in water that is only chest to shoulder deep. This allows for wider participation than in other, more specialized aquatic programs.

Water Exercise Is for Everyone!

Water exercise's popularity also is enhanced by the fact that it can be performed by people of all ages and fitness levels. Most classes offered in aquatic facilities attract young and old, thin and overweight, athletic and sedentary, male and female, and healthy and injured people—and all can participate in the same class! This is possible because the water can accommodate a wide spectrum of movement abilities, permitting each participant to exercise at his or her own pace. Although you might teach your class at an average intensity level, each person can adjust the workout pace to suit his or her needs.

Recently classes with special themes have emerged that are aimed at people with similar interests. Some example are classes for people at high fitness levels (sometimes called *high-energy* classes); for athletes who wish to improve their physical conditioning for sports performance; for patients rehabilitating from an injury or surgery and who require supervision; and for people who have specific chronic medical problems such as multiple sclerosis, cardiac conditions, or arthritis. The YMCA has already recognized the special use of water exercise for those with arthritis by creating the Arthritis Foundation YMCA Aquatic Program in conjunction with the national Arthritis Foundation.

To deal with different types of populations, you may want to read Part III of the accompanying text to this instructor's guide, *Y's Way to Water Exercise*. It covers the different kinds of people—from weight-conscious to performance-minded, from pregnant to aging—who might enroll in your exercise class.

The YMCA and Water Exercise

Water exercise is not new to the Y; it has been a part of Y aquatics programs for many years. The YMCA of the USA has traditionally supported water exercise as a good means for its members to improve their overall physical fitness, part of the Y's goal to help their development of their total human potential. The Y's first water exercise program was outlined in the 1982 book *Physical Fitness Through Water Exercise*. Used by many local YMCAs, this water exercise program became a successful program offering. With the addition of the new *Y's Way to Water Exercise* and this instructor's guide, the YMCA renews its commitment to water exercise and makes a significant contribution to the field.

The YMCA is coordinating this exercise program with other YMCA fitness programs. Although land-based fitness programs and aquatic programs have developed independently, the present Y philosophy is to give all fitness programs a common educational and administrative base. Thus, the Y's Way to Water Exercise program reflects the basic teachings and fitness goals presented in *The Y's Way to Physical Fitness*.

This program, like all other YMCA programs, is designed to help individuals and families grow in many ways:

- It encourages people to set personal goals and to work toward them through well-planned programs.
- It develops the specific skills that aid people in reaching personal goals and improving their self-confidence and self-esteem.
- It provides opportunities for participants to reflect upon their personal values and to better integrate these values into their daily lives.
- It helps people develop cooperative attitudes and effective communication with others.
- It promotes appreciation of diversity of thought, culture, religion, and ethnic tradition, which in turn leads to better understanding and communication among all people.
- It provides opportunities for individuals to become both better leaders and better followers. Shared leadership and support are basic ideas that are taught and practiced in Y programs.

- It fosters fun and enjoyment. Laughter is an essential part of every Y program.

Other YMCA educational programs that might be of interest to participants in water exercise classes include these:

- *The Y's Way to a Healthy Back*—This program combines exercise and instruction on back care to help those who suffer with lower back problems due to loss of flexibility, loss of abdominal strength, poor posture, or excessive tension.
- *Y's Way to Weight Management*—This sensible approach to weight control incorporates education, behavior modification, motivation, and sensible goal setting. For the many people in water exercise classes who want to lose weight, this would be a natural addition.
- *You & Me, Baby*—Pregnant women in your water exercise classes might enjoy becoming involved in this program of prenatal and postpartum fitness classes.
- *Y's Way to Strength Training*—Some class members may want to go from your water exercise class to the weight room to continue working out. Beginners can start with the strength-training book *Building Strength at the YMCA*.
- *Y's Way to Stress Management*—People in your class who are using exercise as a way to reduce stress might be interested in learning more through this balanced program that teaches stress-reduction skills for daily life. It includes managing stress and change; developing a stress-management style; learning personal-management, relationship, and outlook skills; promoting physical stamina; and outlining a management plan.
- *Y's Way to Better Aerobics*—Participants who like to exercise to music can take part in choreographed aerobic exercise classes. If you have an aerobic instructor at your YMCA, you may be interested in *Movin' to Music*, a video/instructional guide package released four times a year. Each package demonstrates a completely new routine and includes 13 or 14 45 r.p.m. records with new music for that routine.
- *Arthritis Foundation YMCA Aquatic Program*—This is a recreational warm-water exercise program designed for anyone suffering from arthritis. Full details on exercises and class organization are available from the *Instructor's Manual*.

The Y's Way to Water Exercise Program

The Y's Way to Water Exercise program is an adaptation of the HydroRobics water exercise program developed at Georgia State University.

The YMCA selected this program because it has been utilized successfully at aquatic facilities around the country and is in tune with the Y's philosophy of physical fitness.

The program was developed over a 10-year period to evaluate all its aspects and be sure it took into account the needs and interests of people of all ages and fitness levels. A basic set of exercises was designed to help each person improve the various components of physical fitness.

Offering a fitness program that appeals to an ever-larger segment of the population is in concert with the Y's objective to involve as many members as possible in physical activity as one means of helping them fulfill their human potential for mind, body, and spirit. The Y's Way to Water Exercise program expands and enhances the overall physical fitness program offerings of the Y, making more choices available to Y members. Because water exercise has been proven to be an excellent substitute for other forms of physical activity, many people use it as a supplement to (or a replacement for) their current personal fitness programs. They find that this approach adds variety to their usual training regimens.

Unique Features of the Program

Certain features of the Y's Way to Water Exercise program distinguish it from others. For one thing, the majority of the exercises are performed *under water*. This means that the muscles must work against the water's resistance; exercising with resistance helps people make fitness gains more quickly.

Another feature of this program is that each exercise works on the muscles in several different ways simultaneously. For example, in doing the Double Leg Lift, a middle body exercise, the arms perform static muscle work in supporting the body while the abdominal and hip muscles perform dynamic types of movement.

Last, the names of the exercises were chosen to be both appealing and descriptive of the exercises. This feature makes it easier for participants to learn and remember the exercises.

The Water Exercises

The specific exercises used in the program (which are described in the text *Y's Way to Water Exercise*) are grouped either by the specific section of the body they are designed to work or by their aerobic affect. Grouping exercises by sections of the body—upper, middle, or lower—allows people who like to emphasize the development of specific areas to easily select those exercises they want to use more often. For instance, someone who wants to tone muscles in the midsection would simply choose more exercises from the middle body group. All these exercises will develop muscular strength, endurance, and flexibility.

The aerobic exercises make up most of the water exercise workout. This portion of the workout lasts from 20 to 30 minutes and is the foundation of the Y's Way to Water Exercise program. These exercises are essential, as they are aimed at improving the heart, the most important muscle in the body. Aerobic exercises also help the participant lose weight, as they demand increased expenditure of calories.

All the exercises have been checked for safety. No exercise that might be harmful to healthy adults has been included. Every exercise that could possibly harm a participant with a physical problem has a specific precaution listed so that you may warn and instruct the participant. For instance, a lower back exercise that causes the back to be slightly arched may be contraindicated for someone who has a back problem.

The Y's Way to Water Exercise Text

Y's Way to Water Exercise is an excellent asset to this water exercise program. The book provides you as an instructor with the body of knowledge you need to teach the course and provides participants with materials that give them insight into the various principles of training and fitness. The book's informal style, clear structure, and detailed fitness information should make it enjoyable reading. The diagrams that accompany the exercise descriptions make the exercises easy to learn and emphasize proper form.

Use by You

Y's Way to Water Exercise is the official text for the YMCA water exercise program. It contains all the exercises recommended for the program. It also can serve as an excellent review of water exercise and fitness information. In addition, you can enhance your teaching by assigning students readings that correspond to the minilectures you give on fitness topics. (Minilectures and reading assignments are discussed in chapters 4 and 6.)

If this is the first time you have taught water exercise, this book will be extremely helpful. Used wisely, it can be the glue that bonds the class and you together to produce a successful exercise experience.

Use by the Participants

We strongly recommend that your participants have copies of this book. Most participants welcome a book to go with their program, especially because it presents details of the exercises and fitness information. The participants might want to use the book to study and work out further on their own, even after they have completed the class. They also need the book in order to participate in the reading assignments. By the way, don't hesitate to make such assignments because you are afraid people will see them as extra work. If you present such assignments in a positive manner—stressing the interesting aspects of the topics and how they apply to students personally—the students soon feel that they miss out on something if they *don't* read the assignments.

You've now learned about the beginnings and growth of water exercise, its advantages, and the Y's special program. In the next chapter we'll discuss how water exercise differs from land-based exercise and what research says about water exercise and fitness development.

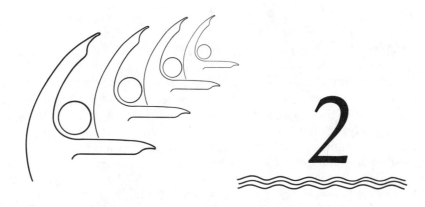

Advantages and Effectiveness of Water Exercise

One of the first questions asked about water exercise is "Can you really get a good workout in the water?" The answer is yes. However, for a good workout, you must take into account and take advantage of the unique properties of water and their effects on exercise physiology and movement. Then, as with any exercise mode, you must adhere to general training principles. Particularly in regard to the development of cardiorespiratory fitness (also known as cardiovascular or cardiopulmonary fitness), research has shown that water exercise is often at least as good as more traditional forms of aerobic exercise, such as running, cycling, or swimming, which may not be the exercise mode of choice for a particular person.

In this chapter we'll discuss the properties of water—buoyancy, resistance, and temperature—that make it a favorable medium for exercise. Research supporting the validity of water exercise is also presented. The next chapter covers physical fitness concepts and how to apply them to your water exercise class.

Water's Effects on Exercise

Exercising in the water is a much different experience than exercising on land. You might like to tell your water exercise participants that exercising in the water is often compared to doing aerobics in outer space, where weightlessness makes movement easier. Because water's *buoyancy* makes the submerged portion of a person's body 90 percent lighter than on land, this analogy is fairly realistic. On the other hand, in order to make water exercise sufficiently intense for participants to achieve fitness benefits, you must teach them how to subvert water's buoyancy and instead work against water *resistance*. Before participants have to deal with these factors, though, the physical characteristic of water that they will probably feel first (besides its wetness, of course) is its *temperature*. (All these characteristics are also discussed in chapter 2 of *Y's Way to Water Exercise*.)

Temperature

Because most pools and bodies of water are cooler than the human body, a person entering the water feels the effects of a transfer of heat from the body (98.6°F) to the water (usually 78°F to 84°F). Of course, the coolness of the water is one of the major attractions of water exercise—in 90° weather with 95 percent humidity, would you rather pound the pavement or jog in the pool? This coolness may make some people uncomfortable initially, but the discomfort is easily overcome if they perform a few warm-up exercises in the water. Encourage your participants to move around as soon as they enter the water.

The coolness of the water may be one of the reasons that a lower maximal heart rate is often found in maximal oxygen uptake tests done in swimming compared with walking. Some fitness proponents, such as Howley and Franks (1986), have suggested that the training heart rate range for water exercise is different from that predicted for land exercise. This will be discussed further in the next chapter.

As an instructor, you should be aware that immersion in cool water can cause a small drop in the body core temperature, even during exercise. The body tries to defend itself against this drop in temperature by shivering. People often find this sensation uncomfortable. In a study reported in 1981, Claremont, Reddan, and Smith found that the body core temperatures of their elderly participants dropped about 1°F after an exercise session in 81°F water lasting about 30 minutes.

They found that complaints about coldness became increasingly frequent after about 20 minutes.

Occasionally, the water might be so warm that heat transfer from the body to the water medium cannot take place. You should realize that exercise in water that is this hot poses the same risks as exercise in hot air—fatigue and heat exhaustion.

Buoyancy

The buoyant force of water may make some exercises easier, but it also makes exercise safer for some people, especially those who are prone to joint problems. The water is a nonweight-bearing, reduced-impact environment. Water exercise is thus ideal for the elderly, overweight, pregnant, or previously sedentary individual. Although this particular Y program does not focus on the rehabilitative advantages of water exercise, the person recovering from injury may find this kind of class helpful in maintaining fitness without exacerbating the injury. All these reasons for joining a water exercise class hold for normal, healthy fitness buffs as well—they too can benefit from the reduced stress on the joints due to water's buoyancy.

Resistance

Water resistance causes a drag effect on limbs when they are moved through the water so the muscles have to work harder to move them. The amount of drag generated is determined by, and appears to be proportional to, the force the limbs exert (their speed) as they move. Therefore, water resistance can provide quite a challenge during cardiovascular fitness, muscle strength, and muscle endurance activities.

Let's look at an activity you might try with your class to demonstrate the effects of water resistance in aerobic activities. Ask the participants to jog slowly in knee-deep water for about 2 minutes, then to jog slowly in midthigh-deep water for the same length of time, then to move as fast as possible in midthigh-deep water. They'll find that each exercise is more difficult than the one before; this is because the resistance increases.

To demonstrate the role of resistance in muscle strength development, have your participants stand in neck-deep water, their arms extended out to their sides. Ask them to lower their arms to their sides, first slowly, then (starting again from the extended position) quickly. They will find that it's more difficult to lower their arms quickly and forcefully because of the water's increased resistance to faster moving objects. For other examples illustrating resistance, see chapter 4.

The Water Exercise Environment

For many people, water is a very pleasurable exercise environment not only because of the obvious physical characteristics of coolness and buoyancy but also because of less obvious and environmental ones. Wave movement creates an overall massage—certainly a pleasure. The whole environment of water exercise is stress reducing. There are probably fewer distractions at the pool than in other exercise settings. For example, a jog down the street might bring an encounter with a ferocious dog or an inconsiderate bicyclist; no such distractions can be found at the pool. There are many other qualities of exercising in water that participants find enjoyable; ask your class what they think.

Research on Water Exercise

The sheer enjoyability of water exercise may be reason enough to enroll in or teach such a class, but in addition, research has shown that water exercise is a very valid fitness activity. The cardiorespiratory benefits are well established. Unfortunately, studies on the effects of water exercise on other measures of fitness—strength, muscle endurance, flexibility, and body composition—have not been done. The technology necessary for some of the required measurements is now in the early stages of development (Koszuta, 1986). As for other measures of fitness, it can only be assumed that adherence to training principles results in improvement.

To determine cardiorespiratory benefits, some studies on water exercise compare walking or jogging in water to the same activity on land. There are even studies that compare cycling in the water with cycling on land! You may initially react by questioning the relationship of these findings to what goes on in your water exercise class—after all, you and your group twist, lunge, do the can-can, and perform jumping jacks, as well as walk or run in the water. However, researchers can objectively determine the effects of the exercise medium (air or water) on physiological responses more easily by studying standard activities rather than by trying to compare the different types of activities unique to each medium.

To see what effects water has on physiological parameters (for example, heart rate and oxygen uptake) during exercise, one approach is to have subjects walk at the same rate on land (on a treadmill) and in water and compare the results. In a recent study reported in 1987 using this approach, researchers Whitley and Schoene found that heart rate, a measure of exercise intensity, increased 135 percent from resting level to the highest walking speed in waist-deep water (about 2.0 mph), whereas the increase in air was only 19 percent. They also found that their subjects, 12 healthy female college students, achieved sufficient intensity for cardiorespiratory benefits (75 percent of predicted maximal heart rate) at a speed of 1.66 mph, a speed that did not produce a sufficient intensity response in air.

An earlier study by Evans, Cureton, and Purvis (1978) looked at oxygen uptake (a measure of caloric expenditures), as well as heart rate and other measures, in male subjects during walking and jogging in water and in air. They found that only about half the speed was required during water exercise for the same level of energy expenditure as exercise in the air. Although it was not possible to accurately determine the percentage of maximal heart rate that the reported heart rates represented, it appeared that walking in the water at a speed of 1.9 mph, which produced an average heart rate of 143 beats per minute, would be in the training heart rate range. From these two studies it is clear that fitness benefits can be gained in water without moving at fast speeds and without actually swimming.

It is clear that walking and jogging in water provide good workouts, but what about activities like those in the Y's water exercise program? Vickery, Cureton, and Langstaff (1983) measured both heart rate and oxygen uptake during a water exercise program called Aqua Dynamics (without comparison to land-based exercises). These researchers found that both the heart rate and oxygen uptake responses indicated that the workouts, consisting of calisthenics and swimming, were of sufficient intensity for cardiorespiratory conditioning according to American College of Sports Medicine guidelines (1978).

Another question that research has addressed concerns types of people for whom water exercise is appropriate. Subjects in the studies so far discussed were young to middle-aged, and it seems that water exercise was indeed appropriate for them. Lloyd, Thiel, Holloman, Fletcher, and Fletcher (1986) described a water exercise program that could be safely used in cardiac rehabilitation programs. Claremont, Reddan, and Smith, in a 1981 study on the feasibility of water exercise programs for the elderly, found that water exercise involving walking at various water depths with and without flutterboards or armstrokes provided a sufficient exercise stimulus for cardiorespiratory conditioning.

Water exercise of some type is often recommended for pregnant women. In a study by McMurray, Katz, Berry, and Cefalo in 1988, the metabolic response of women to water exercise during pregnancy was found to be different from that seen when they were not pregnant, 8 to 10 weeks after delivery. However, this difference was not seen as deleterious, and the authors did not recommend avoidance of water exercise during pregnancy.

For many people, then, it seems that water exercise is a good, safe choice for an aerobic workout. As mentioned earlier, the effects of water exercise on other aspects of fitness have not been quantified. Considering all the benefits, though, water exercise should always be offered as a fitness option. In the next chapter we'll discuss how fitness training concepts can be applied in water exercise classes.

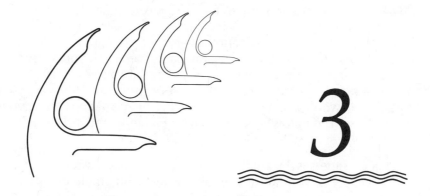

3

Physical Fitness Concepts

Because you are a water exercise instructor, you are probably aware of the necessity of understanding fundamental concepts of exercise physiology in order to teach a safe, effective exercise program. This chapter provides that basic knowledge with particular reference to water exercise programs so that you can feel confident in your teaching and so that you can prepare minilectures for your exercise participants.

In addition to using this material, you should consult with the fitness director at your Y for specific in-house fitness guidelines that may affect your class. Because the general fitness principles of water exercise are the same as those of other fitness classes, you should feel free to consult with other fitness personnel when you have questions about your water exercise class. You'll also find that *Y's Way to Physical Fitness* is an excellent background text for any physical fitness activity class, including one involving water exercise.

Definition of Physical Fitness

Physical fitness means many different things to different people. For one person, being fit means dominating the basketball court; for another, having rippling muscles; for another, getting through a year without a cold; and so on. Because your participants come into your class with so many different preconceptions, it's a good idea to establish a definition of physical fitness very early in your program. This way, your participants won't retain (or form) unrealistic expectations about your fitness class. The following definition by H. Harrison Clarke (1979) is one that we suggest you offer:

> Physical fitness is the ability to carry out everyday tasks with vigor and alertness, without undue fatigue and with ample energy to engage in leisure time pursuits and to meet above average physical stresses encountered in emergency situations. (p. 1)

Point out to your participants that this definition doesn't promise improvements in sport performance, physical appearance, or health as consequences of being physically fit. In particular, they should understand that physical fitness is not the same thing as health; instead, it is one component of good health.

What the definition doesn't address is how to become physically fit. The most important way is through physical activity, including exercise. The following section discusses the ways different kinds of activities—with particular reference to water exercise—promote development of different aspects of fitness.

Components of Physical Fitness

Most fitness experts name the following as being components of physical fitness:

Cardiorespiratory fitness

Body composition

Musculoskeletal fitness, comprising
Flexibility
Muscular strength
Muscular endurance

Although programs that promote the development of a specific component of fitness may be formulated, it is the Y's philosophy to bring together activities in an exercise class that result in some improvement in each component. It is also the Y's philosophy to place the greatest emphasis on cardiorespiratory fitness.

The following sections cover each component of fitness. Chapter 1 of *Y's Ways to Water Exercise* also addresses these issues. You may choose to refer your participants to that book before or while you discuss these components during your class.

Cardiorespiratory Fitness

Cardiorespiratory fitness is often called cardiovascular or cardiopulmonary fitness. Although the terms technically don't mean the same thing, they are often interchanged. No matter which term is used, this aspect of fitness concerns the coordinated effort of the heart (*cardio-*) and lungs (*-respiratory* or *-pulmonary*) to deliver oxygen via the blood vessels (*-vascular*) to working muscles. The muscles need oxygen to use fuels—carbohydrates, proteins (amino acids), and fats—to produce most of the energy needed in low to moderate levels of activity.

Proper breathing is especially important during exercise, so that adequate amounts of oxygen are available. Irregularities in breathing patterns are often common in people who are anxious and nervous. Be aware that your participants may not initially feel comfortable in the water or in an exercise class. Caution your students to avoid hyperventilating (breathing too rapidly) or holding their breath because they could become faint.

For an exercise program to develop cardiorespiratory fitness, most experts recommend that it include *aerobic*, or *endurance*, activities. In 1978 the American College of Sports Medicine (ACSM) issued a statement describing attributes of activities that lead to cardiorespiratory fitness. The activity itself, the ACSM said, should be one that "uses large muscle groups, that can be maintained continuously, and is rhythmical and aerobic in nature (e. g., running-jogging, walking-hiking, swimming, skating, bicycling, rowing, cross-country skiing, rope skipping, and various endurance game activities)" (p. vii). You can see that a water exercise program certainly can be constructed that meets these requirements. The ACSM also makes recommendations concerning the *frequency, intensity,* and *duration* of these activities.

Frequency

How *often* does a person have to exercise to achieve cardiorespiratory benefits? A number of studies indicate that exercise should be performed at least three times a week for cardiorespiratory benefits. Very out-of-shape people do make some initial gains with a two-times-a-week program. The more serious participant, who is looking for more than a basic level of fitness, might work out five or six times a week, often adding or substituting muscular strength and endurance workouts. The Y's water exercise program is based on three workout sessions per week.

Intensity

How *hard* does a person have to exercise to achieve cardiorespiratory benefits? Most researchers agree that a certain threshold of intensity must be exceeded during a session. However, beyond that threshold a range of intensities from moderate to fairly high is advantageous and practical for most people. In your exercise class, intensity is partly controlled by the rhythm of the music—the faster the pace, the higher the intensity (if your participants keep to the beat, of course). However, the forcefulness of the participant's movements also affects intensity; participants have to learn to work against and increase the water resistance, not just letting buoyancy work for them, if they wish to intensify the workout.

Intensity may be expressed in terms of oxygen uptake; this is the measure often used in the exercise science laboratory. The ACSM advises working out at 50 to 85 percent of maximum oxygen uptake. However, measurement of oxygen uptake is not practical in real-world exercise. In the fitness class, intensity is usually gauged by *heart rate* (or *pulse rate*) or *perceived exertion*, which are both related to oxygen uptake.

Heart rate.   As exercise intensity increases, the body must generate more energy, so it must increase its uptake of oxygen. The oxygen, along with the fuels mentioned earlier, is carried in the bloodstream to the muscles, where it is used for energy production. Thus, the heart must pump more blood during exercise to meet the muscles' demand for more oxygen. The heart pumps out more blood by two means: by increasing the amount of blood that is pushed out with each beat, called *stroke volume*; and by increasing the number of beats, or contractions, per unit of time, called *heart rate*. The predominant mechanism of increasing blood and, therefore, oxygen to the muscles during exercise is an increased heart rate. So, the increase in oxygen uptake is reflected in an increase in heart rate. Because of this relationship, we can use heart rate as a measure of how hard the body is working.

We mentioned earlier that exercising within a particular range of intensities seems to lead to cardiorespiratory benefits. This range of intensities, called the *training heart rate range*, may be calculated by taking percentages of the maximal heart rate. The maximal heart rate for a given individual may be precisely obtained by a maximal oxygen uptake test in the lab, or it can be estimated by using this formula:

$$\text{Maximal heart rate} = 220 - \text{age}$$

You can calculate a person's desired training heart rate range as straight percentages of his or her predicted maximal heart rate. This is the method suggested in *Y's Way to Physical Fitness*, where the recommended range is 65 to 85 percent of the predicted maximal heart rate. (This differs slightly from the participant's text, *Y's Way to Water Exercise*, which recommends 60 to 85 percent.) This method gives you a conservative estimate of the training heart rate range; the heart rates obtained by this method tend to be slightly lower than those that would be obtained in the lab. Nevertheless, it's an easy, unintimidating formula that may be especially appropriate for beginning exercisers, who need not be too concerned about exercise intensity during their first few sessions.

Another method for estimating a training heart rate range is the *heart rate reserve method*, originally formulated by Karvonen, a Finnish exercise researcher. The estimated heart rate range derived by this method is more consistent with the one that would be obtained in a lab test. This method is described in chapter 5 of *Y's Way to Water Exercise*.

Some researchers have suggested that the recommended training heart rate ranges may overestimate the training intensity needed for water exercise. Evans, Cureton, and Purvis, in their 1978 study on physiological responses to water exercise, suggest that water temperature affects the training heart rate range. In water cooler than about 80°F, the threshold heart rates obtained using the formulas presented earlier may be too high. Howley and Franks (1986) suggest lowering the training heart rate range by about 10 beats for aquatic activities (if your pool is warm enough, it may not be necessary to make these adjustments). The possibility that the calculated training range is not accurate for water exercise is one reason that it is not advisable for you as the instructor to push a participant to perform at a level that he or she does not find acceptable.

Perceived exertion.   Most people eventually acquire or already have the ability to determine whether or not they are working out hard enough. Ask your participants to become aware of the different sensations as they exercise. As the intensity of exercise increases, they'll notice that breathing and talking become more difficult and fatigue begins to set in. Actually, these perceptions of exertion are closely tied to the physiological processes of fatigue in the body; in the exercise lab, it has been found that subjective self-ratings of exertion increase with objective measures of exercise intensity such as oxygen uptake and heart rate. So, with experience, it is possible for a person to settle into his or her training heart rate range simply according to perceived exertion.

Numerical scales of perceived exertion have been set up, but a less formalized one is often more practical. A good perceived exertion indicator for an aerobic workout is for the participant to exercise to the point where he or she can just barely maintain a "light" conversation with another participant. This effect usually occurs at about 60 percent of the maximal heart rate.

In your class have your participants stop to take their pulse count (using the method described in chapter 4) when they feel as though they are working hard enough. This will help them learn the relationship between perceived exertion and heart rate. For beginning exercisers, the rating of perceived exertion will probably be high and will not correspond to the level of intensity indicated by the pulse, which may not even be in the training heart rate range. Over time, though, participants should become able to estimate their pulse rate during exercise just by the way they feel.

Remember, the maximal heart rate and training range formulas you use are just estimates; the true maximal heart rate may be higher or lower than the estimates. Also, some people never exercise at an adequate level of intensity because they have a low threshold of pain. Encourage your participants to challenge themselves—but again, don't try to force anyone to exercise at a level that he or she feels is unsafe.

Duration

How *long* should the cardiorespiratory (aerobic) portion of the exercise session be? Although anywhere from 15 to 60 minutes of aerobic activity have been suggested in research results, the usual recommendation is 20 to 30 minutes. This is the length of time allocated to aerobic activities in the Y's Way to Water Exercise program, with the remainder of the hour-long class being devoted to development of other fitness components.

Body Composition

The body consists of many components, including bone, muscle, fat, blood, nerves, and organs. Body composition may be conveniently divided into *lean body mass* and *fat mass*. Lean body mass refers to all body tissues except fat. The amount of fat in the body is usually expressed as a percentage of total body weight. Your students are no doubt concerned about body composition because it has a lot to do with physical appearance; a person who has a large percentage of body fat looks unshapely. More importantly, fat adds unhealthy stress on the cardiorespiratory and musculoskeletal systems.

A person who has more muscle tends to perform daily activity with more ease. Because muscle tissue is more metabolically active than fat tissue, that is, muscles burn more calories, a more muscular person is better able to control weight. (Also see chapter 7 on weight management and nutrition.)

A simple test can be conducted by your students if they wish to get a rough idea of whether they are too fat. Simply ask them to pinch and pull away a skinfold from the lower portion of the upper arm, about 2 inches up from the elbow, when the arm is hanging straight down. If the skinfold is more than an inch thick, they should consider themselves as having too much fat. Your Y fitness director could probably arrange for a more accurate test of fat percentage because most Ys have the necessary instrument (calipers) to measure skinfolds. The normal range of percentage of fat is 16 to 20 for men and 19 to 23 for women, depending on age.

Many of your participants will want to know how to lose fat. The best way seems to be through a sensible diet and exercise. The best kind of exercise to promote fat loss is aerobic exercise. The ACSM, in their position paper issued in 1978, suggested that persons interested in fat loss should exercise at least three times a week in sessions that each use up about 300 calories or four times a week in exercise sessions that use up about 200 calories. The caloric expenditure of the Aqua Dynamics water exercise program discussed in the previous chapter was about 200 calories. Thus, it appears that a properly constructed water exercise program provides body composition benefits.

If losing fat while retaining lean body mass has a desirable effect on body composition, it follows that increasing lean body mass without gaining fat would have a comparable effect. Gains in lean body mass can best be achieved, especially for men, through muscular strength activities, which we'll discuss later in this chapter.

Flexibility

Flexibility, one component of musculoskeletal fitness, is the capacity of joints to move through a full *range of motion*. The range of motion is the arc of movement a limb and joint can make within a particular plane. A demonstration of the range of motion of the shoulder joint in the sagittal plane (dividing the body into right and left halves) would be reaching the arm above the head, moving it backward as far as possible, then bringing the arm back forward and downward in an arc to brush by the hip, extending it down and backward as far as possible.

Although a person may be generally described as being either flexible or "tight," flexibility, as you can see in the previous example, is specific to each joint of the body. For example, a person who is flexible for some movements at the hip joint isn't necessarily flexible at the ankle joints. Muscles, ligaments, tendons, and other connective tissue determine the amount of flexibility at each joint, and the way these tissues are organized around bone is largely inherited. However, flexibility can be improved within these genetic limits by moving the joint through its full range of motion during activities and through stretching.

Stretching exercises are often divided into two types, static and ballistic. Static stretching involves moving a selected limb through a predetermined range of motion to be held at a maximum stretch point for 12 seconds or longer. For best results, the movement and hold is repeated several times. A good guideline for determining how far to stretch is the first sign of pain; the position just short of pain should be held. Ballistic stretching involves bouncing (rather than holding) at the end of the range of motion. In general, ballistic stretching is not recommended. If ballistic stretches are to be included, though, use them only after static stretches have been completed. Ballistic stretches may lead to abnormal stretching of muscles, compensatory contraction (shortening) of muscles, a decrease in flexibility, and even injury if they are not carefully performed.

Because maintaining good flexibility will help your students avoid injury and muscle soreness, you'll want to include flexibility exercises and stretches in the warm-up and cool-down portions of your class. Because flexibility is joint-specific, you should include flexibility exercises for most of the joints of the body. You should also encourage joint movement through the full range of motion whenever possible in the other portions of your class.

Muscular Strength and Endurance

Most of your students will be interested in developing their muscles during your water exercise class; almost everybody wants to feel that his or her body is toned rather than flabby. Toning can be achieved through muscular strength and muscular endurance activities, which promote musculoskeletal fitness.

Muscular strength is important in performing everyday tasks, so it need not be associated with lifting 300-pound barbells. For research purposes, *strength* is defined as the maximum amount of force that can be exerted by a muscle. The usual test of strength is to determine how much weight can be lifted one time. However, most people are interested in a more everyday level of strength—they need to lift bags of groceries, 3-year-old nephews, shovelfuls of garden dirt—so testing and training for maximal strength are not necessary.

Strength is developed by subjecting the muscles to an *overload*, a weight or resistance that challenges the muscles. (The concept of overloading is explored in detail later in this chapter.) To take a prosaic example, say you can easily lift a bucket containing 6 pounds of gravel from knee level to shoulder level 10 times. To overload your muscles, you would need to lift more than 6 pounds—perhaps 8 pounds—10 times to develop more strength.

In the example, the pull of gravity on the bucket of gravel offers resistance to your muscles. In water exercise, the water itself offers the resistance, a point discussed briefly in the previous chapter. In the water, your students need to forcefully move against the water. These forceful movements will be met by the resistance of the water, which provides overload *if the participants are moving fast enough* (remember, buoyance can allow some cheating). Your participants need to adjust the speed of their movements so that the muscles are challenged sufficiently for strength development.

Another factor to consider is that strength gain is specific to the angle at which the muscles are exercised. If complete development of the muscle is desired (the Y's water exercise program is designed for this), movements must be performed at several different angles.

In the section on body composition we alluded to the fact that men generally increase their lean body mass through strength activities more easily than women. When discussing strength development, point out to your students that women do not usually build bulky muscles with strength training because most women do not have enough androgens (male hormones) for this bulking to occur. Women who participate in moderate strength-training programs can achieve significant strength improvements with less muscle enlargement than usually occurs in men.

Muscular endurance is the ability of a muscle to exert force repeatedly over a period of time. To return to the previous example: If you could fairly easily lift the bucket with 6 pounds of gravel 10 times, you could challenge your endurance (i.e., you would create an overload) by lifting the same bucket about 15 times, to the point of fatigue. In water exercise, your participants need to set their movement at a moderate speed and increase the number of repetitions of that movement if they want to improve their muscular endurance.

Many people consider muscular endurance a very practical component of fitness, probably more practical than strength. Think of how many low-strength activities require muscular endurance: painting a wall, stirring cake batter, hammering nails, even typing a letter. Keep in mind, and point out to your participants, that increased muscular endurance for particular movements in water does not automatically translate into improved performance of other endurance tasks (see the discussion of specificity in the next section).

Principles of Training

The Y's water exercise program incorporates the basic principles of training that have proven to develop all components of physical fitness most effectively. Some of these principles were mentioned in previous sections of this chapter. In the following section we will treat each training principle systematically. Consider these principles of training in planning and conducting the water exercise program.

Overload

Fitness components most affected:
  cardiorespiratory and musculoskeletal fitness

To make improvements in a particular fitness component, an *overload* must be applied. The physiological systems involved in a particular component must be subjected to a greater workload, or more physiological stress, than they normally encounter. The degree of overload depends on three primary factors: frequency, intensity, and duration. Overload varies according to how these factors are changed, either independently or in combination.

As mentioned earlier, in water exercise, intensity overload for the cardiorespiratory and strength components is created mainly by increasing the speed of movement. It also can be adjusted by planning exercises to reflect how Newton's three laws of motion apply in water.

1. *Law of inertia.* Because force must be applied to change the direction of a body in motion, frequently asking students to change direction of movement will increase the intensity of the workout. Starting, stopping, and restarting in a new direction takes work. For example, instead of having students perform the Joggernaut exercise in place, have them do it forward and backward or side to side.
2. *Law of acceleration.* The distance an exerciser covers and the energy he or she expends to get there will depend on how strong

that person is (how much force that person can exert) and how heavy he or she is. For instance, in the Downhiller exercise a stronger, better conditioned person would be able to jump a greater distance than a weaker, less fit person. Also, a heavier person would use more energy than a lighter person to cover the same amount of distance. This should be taken into account in class planning for less fit students so the pace or distance covered is not greater than they can handle.

3. *Law of action and reaction.* Exercises that require change of direction, such as Downhiller and Side Leg Side, are examples of this law. When the legs move in one direction, the upper body tends to move in the opposite direction. Such movement brings the water's resistance into play, increasing the overload.

Exercises in which the body stays in place are also examples of this law. In Jumping Jacks, the arm and leg on one side of the body move in one direction while the arm and leg on the other side move in the opposite direction. The movements offset each other, causing the body to remain in place.

In the case of muscular endurance, the increasing number of repetitions is the means to increase overload. The section "Exercise Intensity" in chapter 4 contains techniques you can use to get your participants to work with overload.

Specificity

Fitness components affected:
cardiorespiratory and musculoskeletal fitness

The principle of specificity states that the type of gain achieved relates to the type of workout performed. It follows from this principle that if you want to reach a certain level of performance in a specific action (or function) of a particular muscle group (or fitness component), you must practice that specific action during training. For instance, if you want your legs to flutterkick faster in the pool, you have to push yourself to flutterkick faster; you wouldn't do water exercises that strengthen your legs and necessarily expect a faster flutterkick from the generalized strengthening. Likewise, if you want to improve your strength, you should do a strength workout, not an endurance or cardiorespiratory one. It's wise to remind your participants of the principle of specificity.

Progression

Fitness components affected:
cardiorespiratory and musculoskeletal fitness

Once the body or a particular muscle has adapted to a given workload, it must then be subjected to an even greater workload if further improvement is desired. In the case of developing flexibility, progression occurs by slightly increasing the stretch (but never to the point of pain). This process of increasing the challenge, adapting to that challenge, then going on to the next challenge is called *progression*.

Realize that it takes time for adaptation to occur and that people adapt at different rates. Therefore, you must be careful in adjusting the challenges for your class. In general, you should progress when most members of your class have adapted to a particular level of work. As much as possible, suggest challenges that allow for individual differences.

Frequency, Intensity, and Duration

Fitness components affected:
cardiorespiratory and musculoskeletal fitness

Your class's progression is achieved by your increasing the frequency, intensity, or duration of exercise, or some combination of these factors. These factors were discussed earlier, in the section dealing with cardiorespiratory fitness; now we see them applied to other aspects of fitness. When designing a fitness program, you must determine how often (frequency), how hard (intensity), and how long (duration) each exercise or activity should be.

Frequency

An exerciser should work out at least three times a week. This seems to be the general rule for improving cardiorespiratory and musculoskeletal aspects of fitness, and the Y's water exercise program is based on this.

Intensity

Intensity must be adjusted to provide the proper degree of overload.

Duration

The duration range recommended for cardiorespiratory fitness was discussed earlier; the duration ranges for developing other aspects of fitness are not so easily specified. The Y's water exercise program allocates

60 minutes for the entire workout, of which 20 to 30 minutes is directed to cardiorespiratory, aerobic fitness. Gradually increased exercise duration is built into the program: The first few classes use portions of the hour for administrative duties, lecture time, and exercise teaching and demonstration; later on, this time is given over to lengthier aerobic work.

Retrogression

Retrogression is the slowing of fitness gains that often takes place after a few weeks of exercise. During the first phase of a fitness program, gains are rapid and relatively large; later, the gains are smaller. Retrogression is normal and common, but sometimes difficult for the participant to accept. Some people are likely to drop out when retrogression occurs. You can help by offering encouragement and support.

Personalizing the Program

Not everyone responds to exercise in the same way. Some may lose inches from their waists and thighs, others may fatigue less during aerobic activity, and others may simply feel better. People are able to progress and achieve the benefits of exercise at different rates and to different degrees. As an instructor, you should make the participants of your water exercise class aware that individual differences in adjusting to exercise do exist. As mentioned earlier, you may need to suggest modifications in your class, challenges that allow each student to exercise at his or her own level.

In this chapter, we reviewed basic concepts of physical fitness and their applications to water exercise. The next chapter gives you specific information on a variety of techniques to help you become an effective instructor.

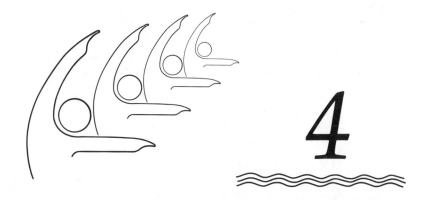

Teaching Methodology

4

The success of an exercise program depends on several variables: program content and design, facilities, and the instructor. Although the program and facilities are important, the instructor is often the determining factor as to whether an exercise program is successful or not.

Instructor Qualifications

The requirements for being an instructor for the Y's Way to Water Exercise program are that you must

- be at least 17 years old,
- successfully complete the Basic YMCA Aquatic Leadership Course,
- possess a current YMCA Lifeguard Certificate,
- possess a current CPR certification card, and
- successfully complete the Y's Water Exercise Workshop.

It also is recommended that you complete the Y's Way to Physical Fitness Specialist certification.

As an instructor of water exercise, you should have a sound back ground in exercise physiology. You need to fully understand the application of basic exercise training concepts and the various con-traindications to exercise. In addition you should be fully qualified and should always act in a reasonable and prudent manner to create safe conditions for participants. Meeting the above minimum requirements helps you conduct a safe and effective water exercise program.

Profile of a Successful Instructor

Every instructor eventually develops his or her unique teaching style. Teaching style can be broken down into several components; how you integrate these into your class will determine your effectiveness. We have selected the following as the components that lead to successful instruction.

Pleasing Physical Appearance and High Fitness Level

Although physical appearance should not be highlighted as being the most important, many participants are motivated by the hope that they can become as attractive as their instructor. However, instead of emphasizing your physical appearance, you should place more sig-nificance on your physical *fitness*. After all, you must be able to sus-tain the same workout you put your class through. Your high fitness level will strengthen participants' respect for you as a leader.

However, physical perfection is not necessary. A partially overweight or less fit instructor can surmount this physical limitation with positive characteristics, such as an outgoing personality.

Good Voice Quality and Projection

Your commands and instructions must be heard by all participants. Unfortunately, when you teach in a pool environment, this may be hard. Competing noise may come from other classes, lap swimmers, or radios. Some tips for overcoming noise and communicating clearly appear later in this chapter, in the "Teaching Techniques" section.

Good Visual Instruction

Whether you are in the water or on the deck, you should make sure that everyone in your class can clearly see your demonstrations. Tips for this are also in the upcoming "Teaching Techniques" section.

Good Preparation and Organization

You should always allot a specific amount of time before class to organize your program content and teaching plan. Using the lesson plans in this manual will help you orchestrate a successful experience for your class.

Know the sequence of exercises to be taught and the time allocation for each. If you are a new instructor and are less confident of your teaching ability, always have one or two standby exercises to call upon in case you forget your planned routine. This will buy you time to remember the planned exercise sequence.

Also review the material in *Y's Way to Water Exercise* in preparation for discussing the assigned readings. You will be more confident going into your class if you are well-prepared. You will feel highly rewarded when your class gives you a standing ovation to acknowledge a good workout or when individuals compliment you on a job well done.

Thorough Knowledge of the Subject

You must have a thorough knowledge of the subject matter. Although to become a YMCA water exercise instructor you must meet specific knowledge requirements, you need to continually review the theoretical subject matter. This not only helps in answering spontaneous questions from the students, but it also reminds you of proper instructional techniques. Both the participant's book and this instructor's guide will be invaluable to you in such review.

Pleasant Personality

Personality is often considered to be one of the most important characteristics of a successful exercise instructor. A pleasant, outgoing instructor generates excitement and a stronger desire to work hard on the part of students. This type of instructor can motivate participants so exercise is fun, not a chore.

Although being outgoing may be beneficial in teaching, not everyone is an extrovert. If you feel you aren't, the following suggestions may help:

- Be available 5 to 10 minutes before or after class to casually chat with participants. This sets the stage for comments on problems they may be experiencing or other questions they may have.
- Occasionally comment about how well individuals are performing in class.

- Keep a light sense of humor, occasionally joking, to create a comfortable atmosphere and to divert participants from noticing the rigors of a challenging workout.
- Move around frequently when teaching from the water, as many people like an instructor to take an active approach to exercise.
- Offer specific corrections on exercises, with plenty of encouragement, on a one-to-one basis when possible.
- Always be polite and genuinely interested in your students.

These techniques are easily learned and may help even the introverted instructor to appear to be more outgoing. Although you probably can't change your overall personality, you can change specific behaviors. Give it a try!

Steps of Teaching an Exercise

If participants are going to obtain maximum benefits from the water exercise program, they need to learn to perform each exercise properly. To establish good exercise habits early in the sessions, you should allocate sufficient time to teach each exercise. Divide the exercises into small groups and take the first five or six class sessions to teach them. In this way the participants learn proper exercise technique and form while beginning to develop their physiological responses to exercise. As the exercise routine is slowly established, each participant learns to adapt his or her own exercise pace to the class pace.

Each exercise should be taught in the following sequence:

1. *State the name of the exercise.* This helps the participants associate the name with the exercise. (A good learning practice is for the students to restate the name of the exercise after they have performed it themselves.)
2. *Explain which sections of the body and components of fitness are involved in the exercise.* Many people exercise to work on specific parts of the body and want to learn what each exercise does for them. When you explain the muscles involved in an exercise, use their more common names rather than their specific anatomical names. You don't need to impress (or daunt) your students with fancy terms.
3. *Demonstrate the exercise.* Generally demonstrate exercises from the pool deck rather than in the water. This gives the participants a better visual picture and helps them learn much faster. However, be sure to wear foot gear such as tennis shoes or to use a mat when teaching from the pool deck. The following

exercises are best demonstrated in the water: Double Leg Lifts, Modified Scissors Cross, Windshield Wiper, and Universal. Have the class observe from the pool deck while you demonstrate these exercises in the water.

4. *Teach using the part-whole method.* The part-whole method of teaching is often used when teaching physical education and recreation skills. With this method, a complex skill or movement is broken down into simpler elements. You should isolate the upper and lower body movements and teach these independently of each other. Once the class is familiar with each of the movements separately, then show how to combine the movements in a coordinated manner to perform the complete exercise.

The following teaching sequence for the Cross-Country Skier exercise demonstrates the part-whole method:

1. You demonstrate leg movements.
2. Participants practice leg movements.
3. You demonstrate arm movements.
4. Participants practice arm movements.
5. You demonstrate combined leg and arm movements.
6. Participants practice combined leg and arm movements.

While the participants practice the combined or whole movement, you should continue to present specific information about the exercise (e.g., position of hands, straightness of arms, and good posture) to help them refine their performance.

5. *Give exercise precautions when necessary.* When teaching an exercise that is potentially harmful when performed improperly, repeatedly tell your class to perform the exercise with caution. Although none of the exercises in *Y's Way to Water Exercise* is considered to be harmful if performed correctly, certain exercises (especially those involving the lower back) may be harmful if done incorrectly or if done by persons with certain orthopedic or other health conditions. See Chapter 5, "Safety Concerns," for more on danger signs of exercise and exercises potentially harmful to the lower back. Cautions are also listed for specific exercises in *Y's Way to Water Exercise.*

Once your class has learned the exercises, stress performing the exercises with proper intensity. This is necessary if participants are to gain maximum benefits from the exercises. When you teach aerobic exercises, emphasize striving for the training heart rate range and working at a minimum level of 65 percent intensity.

If you take the time to teach the exercises correctly, your class will participate more seriously. They will work harder because you have stressed the importance of exercising properly.

Teaching Techniques

This section presents a variety of teaching techniques that will help you teach water exercise effectively. These techniques have been shown to work.

Exercise Intensity

Participants need to understand exercise intensity (the amount of effort or force generated during exercise) and how to move in the water in order to increase the overload on their working muscles. Water exercise class beginners are apt to perform gliding movements at a slow, comfortable pace during an exercise. This approach is facilitated by the buoyant effect of the water, which tends to make movement easier. Consequently, participants must be taught to speed up their movements and take advantage of the water's resistance. To teach this, have the participants stand in chest-deep water and swing their extended arms along the water's surface through a full range of motion. They should start each motion with their arms extended as far back as possible, then swing their arms forward with their palms open in the direction of the motion. Have them do this several times at what they feel is 100-, 75-, 50-, and 25-percent effort or speed (although each person may have a different comprehension of the various degrees of effort, the variance from others will not be significant).

Continue until the participants can perform the arm movement at about 60 percent of maximal effort. Once they are able to perform at this speed, this intensity training technique may be applied to one exercise from each exercise group (aerobic and upper, middle, and lower body). This session may be supplemented with a short lecture on the meaning of training intensity as it applies to muscular and aerobic development. It may be necessary to repeat this training drill in two or three different class sessions to emphasize the development of this skill; this ensures proper exercise intensity for the remainder of the program. Participants quickly learn to put effort into their exercise routines to obtain the benefits.

So participants can monitor how hard they are working during a workout, teach them how to check their heart rate at rest and during exercise. For most people, the easiest place to find a pulse is at either carotid artery in the neck. Tell your participants to place the index and middle fingers of one hand in the hollow on one side of the Adam's apple; they should lightly slide their fingers in this hollow until they feel the pulse. Caution them that excessive pressure on the carotid can actually cause the heart rate to slow, so, for the sake of accuracy and safety, they should exert only slight pressure.

Participants can find the pulse at the radial artery, on the thumb side of the wrist, with a somewhat similar method. They should slide the index and middle fingers to a point about 1 inch from the wrist joint on the inner part of the forearm.

As the instructor, you should tell the participants when to start and stop taking the 10-second heart rate check. First ask them to find the pulse. When everyone's ready, give them a signal to start the count. The first beat they feel after they hear or see the signal should be counted as "one." Tell them that they should continue counting until the second signal, which you give after 10 seconds. They should then multiply the number they obtained by 6 to get their heart rate (i.e., the number of beats in 10 seconds x 6 = the number of beats in 60 seconds, or 1 minute). If they use this method during or immediately following exercise, they should be able to determine whether they were working at the proper exercise intensity, that is, within the training heart rate range (discussed in chapter 3).

Exercise Form

Form should not be confused with exercise technique. Instead of dealing with the method of movement, the concern now is with the form of movement (e.g., position and alignment of the legs and the arms during exercise). For example, the Cross-Country Skier exercise requires that both arms and legs be relatively straight. In this way, the major muscles in the shoulder, hip, and stomach are utilized. If an individual were to bend at the elbows or knees, though, most of the effect of the exercise would be minimized.

If a participant continues to perform an exercise incorrectly, you can use the following approaches to correct the situation:

- Review the proper technique of the exercise while you stand next to the student having problems. This allows him or her to focus on your instruction, which should include highlighting the improper technique.
- Ask the participant to remain after class. Point out the problem and offer corrective instruction. Consider manually assisting the participant, gradually moving his or her limbs with less force when he or she begins to respond with the correct movement.

Study "The Water Exercises," Part II in *Y's Way to Water Exercise*, to become as familiar with the exercises as possible. Remember to continually stress proper exercise form in class.

Positions During Teaching

Be sure you can be seen at all times, especially when you are teaching an exercise that is new to the class. During the instructional phase, teach most exercises from the pool deck. Once they are familiar with the exercises, most classes enjoy having instructors enter the water to lead exercise periods. Some exercises are more appropriately taught from the water with the class observing from the pool deck. In this case, use the corner of the pool as a teaching station and choose a depth that allows even the shortest student a chance to observe.

Observation

Frequently change your position to obtain a better view of participants; this helps you spot errors and make necessary corrections in form or technique. This is best done from the pool deck. Once you are in the water, it is more difficult to observe your students' underwater movements. Consequently, make as many corrections as possible early in the program, when you are predominantly teaching from the deck.

Communicating Instructions

If your class is to follow your directions, they first need to hear them clearly. Especially when the class is large, your speaking with a loud, commanding voice helps participants follow instructions more easily and gives them the feeling that you are in control. Always face your class when you speak; direct instructions toward the center of the group. Try to project your voice as much as possible. Projecting may be difficult if you have a low-pitched voice. If this is the case, try increasing your volume by taking deeper breaths and actively using your diaphragm. You might also try speaking more slowly so that words sound more distinct.

If all attempts to project your voice fail, you may need to consider using devices such as a bullhorn or a cordless mike. Otherwise, you can try using the technique of *split commands*: Project your commands toward half of the class, then immediately repeat the same commands toward the other half. Although this may become tedious, it is an effective, inexpensive way for you to be sure your students hear your instruction.

Finally, try to cut down on the amount of noise in the pool area. Ask the pool manager to schedule as few other programs and activities as possible during your class hour. Also, have the lifeguards enforce pool noise and horseplay regulations when others share the pool with your class.

Dos and Don'ts of Teaching

You should emphasize the following dos and don'ts of teaching water exercise:

DO	*DON'T*
Select exercises to vary the angles of muscle groups.	Don't overwork specific muscle groups by selecting exercises that work muscles at only one angle or dimension.
Emphasize static stretching techniques.	Don't encourage ballistic, bouncing types of movement.
Encourage participants to relax their feet and toes during exercise.	Don't encourage participants to point toes or arch the feet, because this may lead to cramps.
Encourage proper breathing, which consists of exhaling during expanding movements and inhaling during inward or contracting movements.	Don't ignore breathing coordination. Be concerned about overbreathing or hyperventilation.
Teach the use of proper foot placement, with the heels pushed down, particularly in the aerobic exercises.	Don't let participants land on their toes only, because this may lead to overdevelopment of the calf muscles as well as cramps.
Teach pelvic tilting or abdominal tightening to prevent hyperextension in the lower back (see "Exercise Precautions" in chapter 5 for more on this topic).	Don't teach hyperextension of the lower back. Modest extension may be necessary to strengthen lower back muscles, though.
Promote taking advantage of the physical characteristics of water for strengthening muscles. Participants must move with speed to utilize the water's resistance.	Don't let participants use gliding movements.

(Continued)

DO	**DON'T**
Use a variety of music to please all interests and vary the intensity of the workout.	Don't keep playing the same tape over and over. Furthermore, it is *not* necessary to use music all the time, especially during the early, instructional phase of the class.

Adapting Your Teaching to Pool Conditions

Pool conditions may not always be ideal when you are teaching. The water may be colder than usual, or the pool may not be deep enough to have a gutter or rail for participants to hang on to. Luckily, there are some ways you can adapt your teaching to compensate for these problems.

Cold Water

On many occasions the water temperature may drop below normal. This may be due to mechanical failure of the indoor pool's heating system or abnormal climatic conditions affecting the outdoor pool. In any event, these cooler conditions may affect your class's comfort. It is quite possible that some people may not be able to exercise at all, especially those with health problems that are easily aggravated by cooler temperatures, such as arthritis.

When the water temperature has dropped below the normal comfort range of 78 to 84 °F, change the structure of the workout to include more aerobic activity. This elevates the body's core temperature and makes the workout more tolerable. Intersperse aerobic exercises throughout the upper, middle, and lower body exercises, during which the body tends to cool down. Another warming tactic is to have participants wear T-shirts over their bathing suits. In addition, they can play water games, which tend to take their minds off the cooler temperatures (see the "Water Games" section later in this chapter).

Pool Design

Because of the design of the pool, you may have to adjust portions of the water exercise program. A pool with a maximum depth of 4 feet does not easily provide good aerobic workouts; the water's resistance (and thus, overloading) is lost to upper body movement because most of the chest and shoulders are above water. Classes that are purposely scheduled for the shallow end of a pool also have this problem.

The only solution to a shallow pool is to emphasize exercises and movements that stress the lower body, because that is where the large muscle groups that can be overloaded for aerobic exercise are located. Still, arm movements should continue to be part of exercises; you must attempt to maintain the integrity of each aerobic exercise even if the loss of some upper body benefit is unavoidable.

Another problem is presented when a pool does not have a feature such as a gutter or rail to grip for upper body stabilization. In such a case, several middle body exercises that require upper body stabilization (Double Leg Lifts, Modified Scissors Cross, Six Count Twister, Windshield Wiper) will have to be omitted. You can still conduct a good workout by substituting a number of aerobic and lower body exercises that affect the major muscles in the middle body area such as the stomach, hips, and buttocks. Such exercises include the High Jump, the Cossack With High Kick, Leg Circles (with extra emphasis on a large leg circle), and the Pendulum (with a high leg lift in the forward position). Additional exercises using plastic jugs can supplement the middle body workout (see the "Water Jugs" section later in this chapter).

Additional Class Activities

Because Y classes emphasize learning, cooperation, and fun as well as fitness, they incorporate a number of activities besides exercise routines. The following activities, which are built into the lesson plans in chapter 6, will make your classes educational, lively, and interesting.

Minilectures

Many instructors have had much success with conducting occasional 5- to 10-minute minilectures on a variety of fitness topics before the class enters the water. Experience has shown that participants who have a better understanding of the basic exercise concepts are likely to approach their workouts more seriously and enthusiastically. Suggested minilecture outlines appear in Appendix A of this book.

Because participants in the Y's Way to Water Exercise program are encouraged to obtain the participant's text for the program, you should assign readings to coincide with your minilecture schedule. Then both you and your class can use the minilecture time more effectively. Class members may want to discuss what they know or have just learned about a topic.

Circuit Training

Most water exercise participants enjoy an occasional departure from the normal exercise routine. The traditional use of land circuit-training techniques is quite easily adapted to the water. In this approach, you designate a series of exercise stations, each of which is devoted to a single exercise. A small group of participants performs the exercise at a station for a predetermined amount of time while other groups exercise at other stations. At a given signal, all the groups change stations and perform their new exercises for the set time. This process is repeated until every group has visited every exercise station in the circuit.

This technique may be applied to one or more of the different groups of exercises that make up the Y's Way to Water Exercise program. For example, you could design a circuit for just the middle body exercise group, using all nine exercises and identifying a station for each. A time interval of 1 minute per station might be chosen, with participants performing as many repetitions as possible in that time frame. You could design a circuit-training workout for the entire session, using all of the exercise groups. Appendix B is a sample water exercise circuit for a 50-minute class.

Water Games

Another method of making a water exercise workout more exciting is to introduce water games. Water games add an element of fun and competition without sacrificing the fitness benefits of a good workout. Appendix C is a list of sample water games.

Water Jugs

Several water exercise programs use plastic gallon jugs (milk, juice, or others) in their classes. These jugs are inexpensive if purchased from a local vendor. Many instructors simply ask class members to bring two jugs from home. An excellent middle body workout can be designed that uses water jugs, which can be particularly helpful when a pool provides no gutter or rail for holding on to the wall. These exercises are best done in chest- to shoulder-depth water and simply involve a variety of body movements with the arms extended, holding the jugs. A list of exercises using jugs appears in Appendix D.

Relaxation Techniques

Relaxation techniques are ideally suited to the water. Occasionally allocating 3 to 5 minutes of relaxation during cool-downs may become a special treat for class members. Try the following relaxation exercise.

Call all of the participants toward a corner of the pool. The participants should be facing you while you are positioned in the corner of the pool. Have them space themselves at arm's length in all directions.

Ask the participants to lower their bodies to chin depth and to close their eyes. In a low, soothing voice, ask them to relax with their arms extended in front of their bodies. Throughout the exercise, draw their concentration to the lightness of their arms, which are floating due to the buoyancy of the water. Also repeat the word *relax* throughout.

Have the participants take several deep breaths at intervals throughout the procedure. Tell them to direct any tension in their bodies toward their shoulders, through their arms, and then out through their fingers and into the water. Once the tension is released, allow for a minute of quiet time in this position. In a low voice, suggest concentrating on the movement of the water on their bodies—a soothing feeling. At the end of the relaxation period, have them all take a deep breath and slowly open their eyes as they stand up. Have them repeat the deep breath and exhale as you dismiss them. This really works!

Mental imagery may also be incorporated effectively into this technique. Two examples of mental imagery are (a) picturing yourself lying alone on an island beach at dusk, listening to the sounds of the waves crashing repetitively on the shore and (b) making believe you are an astronaut floating in space, gazing attentively at the stars while enjoying the calm, quiet surroundings. Introduce imagery after the procedure of relaxing and releasing tension has been completed.

Use of Water Exercise Training Devices

Many devices have been developed recently to increase the benefits of water exercise. There are vests that help keep the body floating in a vertical position for deep-water jogging. Another type of vest is designed to hold weights and is used to counter the buoyant forces of the water for a more strenuous workout. There are also hand paddles, webbed gloves, and other two-handed devices that effectively increase the surface area of the arms and hands; these products increase the resistance factor during exercise, thus improving the overload effect on the working muscles.

Although these devices are beneficial, they are not necessary for the average water exercise class. The rationale behind this statement is that the surface area of the human body produces sufficient resistance during exercise to improve fitness to an average or above-average level. Nevertheless, these devices serve a threefold purpose: to be used (a) to develop above-average fitness levels; (b) for physical rehabilitation; or (c) for varying the workout to avoid the monotony of routine workouts.

Although your YMCA may wish to purchase such devices, this increases the expense of your water exercise program. Thus, more thought should be given to swimming aids that may already be available, such as kickboards, hand paddles, and swim fins.

Physical Fitness Testing

At the start of the program, have participants self-administer the physical fitness tests in chapter 5 of *Y's Ways to Water Exercise*. The results will give them a base of reference for gauging their improvement when they test at the end of the program. This set of tests was developed specifically for the water exercise program. Although the tests are similar to those in the Y's Way to Physical Fitness program, their administration and interpretation are somewhat different. They do not replace the more accurate Y's Way to Physical Fitness tests. Because you need to arrange for your Y fitness staff to conduct the skinfold measurement portion of the testing anyway, you might suggest to participants that they take the full Y's Way to Physical Fitness testing battery.

If time permits, testing may be repeated at the midpoint of the class. If a measurable gain is noticed, it will serve as a strong motivational tool for the remainder of the program. When little or no gain is realized, then it is hoped some positive psychological benefit (an improved sense of well-being, more energy, or generally feeling better) may still motivate the student. Encourage a student experiencing little gain to have a positive attitude and to continue exercising. Mention that some people just take longer to respond physiologically to exercise for genetic or other reasons.

Motivation Strategies

One of your most challenging tasks is to motivate your class members to continue to come to class. Remember, half the battle has been won when the participant has moved past the procrastination stage and is attending class.

The problem is that it usually takes 5 to 6 weeks for a person to attain noticeable physiological gains from exercise. Therefore, the first few weeks are critical. It may also be a difficult time for participants because they may be having trouble rearranging their schedules to make time for exercise and may be experiencing some discomfort from the activity. You can help by being aware of the different reasons individual students exercise, then inducing them to continue with appropriate words of encouragement.

Why People Exercise

People are lured to water exercise programs for many reasons. The following are just some of them:

- To lose weight for health reasons or to look better
- To feel better, experiencing more energy and feeling happier
- To contour the body, shaping up muscles in specific areas and losing weight
- For medical reasons, when health problems prevent other forms of exercise
- For fun, especially as a chance to socialize
- As an alternative to other fitness activities

All these reasons are valid. You should remember them when some class members don't seem to keep up with the pace. They may be more concerned with the social or fun parts of the class than the physiological benefits. But you know what? That's okay! They may be getting just what they want from the class right now, and they may find that they enjoy the health benefits as well when their fitness levels increase more noticeably.

Reinforcing Participation

Keep in mind that the things you say to students do make a difference. Always acknowledge participants' efforts when they perform a good workout. You'll find that complimenting the entire class or individuals can give them a motivational high. Complimenting people when they look as if they have begun to firm up or have lost a few pounds is a great incentive. A pat on the back just to recognize someone's effort to attend class regularly—regardless of how hard that person works out—might be the positive gesture that motivates him or her to keep exercising.

Encourage members of the class to compliment each other as well. Don't underestimate peer support!

The final chapter in *Y's Way to Water Exercise*, entitled "How to Stay With It!," offers helpful information about motivating the new class member to stick with exercise. Also, encourage the class to read that chapter to gain a better understanding of the techniques they might use to keep going when their enthusiasm fades.

The numerous teaching suggestions just presented should help you teach. The next chapter encourages you to develop a sensitivity to the safety concerns of the participant. Particular attention is given to exercise precautions and to danger signs that might arise during exercise.

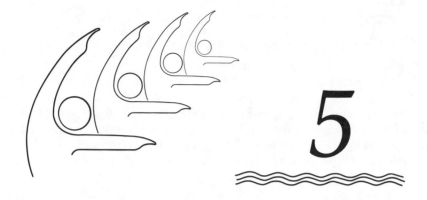

Safety Concerns

As an instructor, you are responsible for the people in your class. You need to take every precaution to prevent injury or harm to them. It may be easy, especially if you are inexperienced, to become so over-zealous in teaching an exercise routine that you overlook the safety of class members. That's why it is extremely important to follow safety procedures in teaching every water exercise class.

Administrative Safety Planning

Administrative duties can sometimes be frustrating. Filling out forms and maintaining records on students is not the favorite part of class for most instructors. However, paperwork is necessary to help protect the health of participants and to document procedures. It is advisable to keep forms and records on file for several years. Check the laws of your state to determine what the statute of limitations is for negligence and contract actions. In addition, emergency procedures must be clearly worked out prior to classes in the event you need to handle an urgent medical problem.

Medical History Forms

A medical history form gives you basic information about your participant's health. This is important because even minor health problems can affect exercise performance. Medical problems can be further complicated by exercise, although the buoyancy of water presents a generally safe exercise environment.

Health screening with a medical history form is an essential first step in your program. A form for your use appears in Appendix E. When the forms are returned, read each one thoroughly. You need to be aware of the physical or medical limitations of each person, even if a doctor has declared him or her healthy enough to participate in a normal exercise class. (However, the doctor determines whether or not a participant should stay *out* of your program because of a health problem—not you!)

Unless you have special medical training, be sure you don't offer any prescriptive advice to participants with health problems. For example, don't prescribe any special exercise routines for remedying particular physical or health conditions. Furthermore, don't discuss how specific individuals should approach their personal diet or nutrition goals, especially if they have had difficulty in the past. Instead, tell them to consult with their personal physicians about their needs and about modifications to their workouts. The only safe advice that you might offer is to suggest that the participant approach the exercise routine in moderation or not do certain exercises at all if they cause too much pain or discomfort.

Once you have reviewed the medical history forms, you may wish to inform individuals with health problems before the first class that you are aware of their conditions. This is the best time to find out what they have discussed with their physicians regarding exercise and exercise restrictions. Also, it is comforting for participants to know that you will be available for further discussion any time problems develop during the exercise program. This approach creates a favorable climate that allows participants to open up and share additional information about their problems as well as to begin their program with enthusiasm.

Ask any participant with a major medical problem to obtain from his or her physician a written note acknowledging the participant's ability to exercise with or without limitations. (A form for this appears in Appendix E.) It is the participant's responsibility to adhere to the limitations, whereas it is your responsibility to establish an overall safe exercise class for *all* participants.

It's best to keep all medical history forms on file in the aquatic office so they are available immediately in case of medical emergency. These forms may give emergency personnel information that will enable them to administer the best possible emergency care.

The following list names health problems that warrant your immediate attention. If any of these problems are noted on a participant's medical history form or if you notice them before a class session begins, recommend to the participant that he or she not enter the water.

- Open wounds
- Infected skin conditions
- Urinary tract infections or cystitis (inflammation of the bladder)
- High fever
- Severe asthma, epilepsy, or angina
- Perforated eardrum
- Severe immobility
- Respiratory infection
- Burns
- Acute sinus infection
- High, low, or unstable blood pressure

For further information about specific health problems, read chapter 13 in *Y's Way to Water Exercise*, "Health Problems: A Panacea?"

Informed Consent Forms

An informed consent form is frequently used in exercise classes. It is intended to make the participant aware of the inherent risks in performing exercise and usually states that the YMCA and its agents assume no liability for injury that may occur during the activity.

Even though the courts may interpret informed consent forms differently in different states, they are valuable documents to have on file. If the form does not include a statement that lists the danger signs that may arise during exercise, participants should be verbally told of these possible adverse reactions to exercise in the first class session. They should be told that in the event that a danger sign occurs, they should stop exercising and bring it to your attention. This guideline may help save a participant from serious harm. (The danger signs that may arise during exercise are listed later in this chapter.)

Although the use of these forms varies greatly between local YMCAs, it is an administrative procedure that every Y director and water exercise instructor should consider. A blank form for your use appears in Appendix E.

Emergency Procedures

Emergency procedures must be designed to bring the quickest and best possible medical assistance to an individual experiencing a medical emergency. All YMCA facilities should have an established, documented emergency protocol. The aquatic director is responsible for seeing that all aquatic staff members are familiar with the emergency procedures.

In the event that water rescue is necessary, the pool lifeguard is primarily responsible for the rescue. If you are playing a dual role as instructor and lifeguard, you should initiate the rescue. In this circumstance, other aquatic staff members should respond by making any necessary phone calls for medical assistance.

Class Safety

Once your water exercise class has begun, you have a definite responsibility to help prevent any injury to participants. This is the time for you to apply all the knowledge you have gained through your training to check for hazards prior to each class session, to competently lead exercises, and to watch participants for medical problems or signs of overexertion.

Equipment and Facility

The pool facility and equipment should be properly maintained. Although the pool and its surroundings are primarily the responsibility of the aquatic director and in-house maintenance staff, you should do a quick inspection of the pool area before each class. Make sure all safety equipment, such as lane markers or signs, is present. Any potential hazards, such as loose tiles, slippery decks or locker room floors, or unusually abrasive pool walls or flooring, should be brought to the attention of the aquatic director immediately.

Proper maintenance of the water chemistry and temperature should be constantly monitored. Air temperature should be about 2 to 4 °F warmer than the water. About 50 to 60 percent relative humidity is ideal.

Water exercise equipment, such as hand paddles, flotation devices (including plastic jugs), and any other commercial devices, is generally your responsibility. Loss or damage of the equipment should be reported to the aquatic director. More expensive and long-lasting equipment, such as tape decks, may require periodic maintenance or repair.

Lifeguard

It is strongly recommended that a qualified lifeguard be on duty during your water exercise class. A lifeguard becomes especially important when a large class (20 or more students) is in session. When teaching in the water, you have limited visibility and cannot see all the students; a lifeguard can watch participants in the back of the group. Also, in case of an emergency, you will have the lifeguard to take charge of the situation.

Exercise Precautions

Participants may injure themselves if you teach exercises improperly. Injury may be immediate, such as a muscle pull or a sprain, or long term, as an injury develops over a period of time. Therefore, you need to fully understand each exercise that makes up the Y's Way to Water Exercise program.

People who have lower back pain must learn to perform the exercises correctly or they risk aggravating their condition. The following are examples of exercises that may place added strain on the lower back if performed incorrectly:

- Body Twist
- Double Leg Lift
- Fire Hydrant
- Six Count Twister
- Windshield Wiper
- Golf Swing
- Quad Stretch
- Pendulum (near-leg movement)
- Cossack Shuffle
- Aerobic exercises involving jumping movements, such as Cheerleader Jump, High Jump, Polaris, and Bunny Hop

A participant who experiences some lower back pain should be advised to perform the movements with *extreme moderation.* Tell him or her to limit the curvature of the spine by tilting the pelvis (bottom forward, top backward). A common expression used is to ask the participant to do "tummy tucks" to cue this position. Tightening the stomach muscles (rectus abdominis) causes the lower back to flatten out. If the participant experiences continued pain from performing an exercise, substitute a familiar exercise from the same group that he or she knows does not cause pain.

When using the training heart rate method of aerobic training, you need to take into account the effect of medications on heart rate. Certain heart or blood pressure medications reduce the heart rate by as much as 10 to 20 beats per minute, depending upon the type of medication and the individual's physiology. For more information, consult "Health Problems: A Panacea?" (chapter 13 in *Y's Way to Water Exercise*), or discuss the effects with your Y's physical fitness director.

Danger Signs During Exercise

A participant experiencing some difficulty during exercise usually shows some sign of distress. You must be able to detect such danger signs when teaching a class. This is extremely important: If participants who are having distress continue to exercise, they may develop much more serious problems. Some of the most important danger signs and their possible causes are listed here:

Sign	*Possible Cause*
Dizziness, shortness of breath, chest or arm pain	Heart problem
Pain in joints	Orthopedic problem, overuse
Muscle cramps	Overuse, lack of sodium or potassium
Reddening of the face	Overwork, heart problem, heat exhaustion
Paleness (face), tiredness, weakness	Heart problem, heat exhaustion
Light-headedness, dizziness, incoherence	Valsalva effect from holding breath too long; hyperventilation
Difficulty breathing	Chronic bronchitis, asthma, overwork, cardiac failure, anxiety
Immersion	Poor balance, slipping, epilepsy, overwork, stroke, heart attack

If you notice any of these signs, unobtrusively motion the affected individual to the side of the pool and ask how he or she is feeling. Usually the person will acknowledge the problem and describe the feeling, at which time you may ask the person to leave the water or to just rest at the side. Continue to monitor the person. If he or she decides to go back to the locker room, make sure a pool staff member accompanies him or her in case a medical emergency arises.

Teaching in a "Prudent and Reasonable" Manner

Being prudent and reasonable in teaching the Y's Way to Water Exercise program means that you take every precaution to ensure that you conduct the program safely. The health and well-being of each participant require that all program procedures be followed routinely, yet carefully. The following is a partial list of dos and don'ts that will help you act in a prudent and reasonable manner.

DO

- Have every class participant fill out a medical history form. Read each form and be familiar with participants' medical problems. Keep the forms available during every class in the event of an emergency.
- Inspect the pool and immediate teaching area both for hazards and obstacles and for missing safety equipment (lane markers, signs, etc.). Correct the problems before class begins.
- Check air and water temperature and pool chemical balance for proper conditions.
- Check to see whether the lifeguard is on duty, if one has been assigned to the class.
- Watch participants for signals of distress during exercise. Assess a potential problem immediately without disturbing the class.
- Recommend that participants who have health-related difficulties with exercise discuss their problem with their physician.
- Teach using only the format recommended in *Y's Way to Water Exercise.*
- Select the proper exercise intensity for participants and never overwork them. Don't encourage them to "go for the burn" and don't badger the less physically fit to work harder. Progressively increase intensity levels only as the majority of participants improve their fitness levels.
- Tell class members to work at their own pace, based on their training heart rate, when doing aerobics.
- Advise participants to listen to their body's signals to prevent injury. When using music or a cadence, teach students with lower or higher fitness levels to adapt to the pace by exercising with slower or faster movements. The fine-tuning procedure helps produce a more individualized and safer workout.
- State specific exercise precautions when necessary (check *Y's Way to Water Exercise* instructions for exercises for specific warnings).

DON'T

- Don't ever make any prescriptive statements to participants with health problems. You may be held liable for any negative results of your advice.
- Don't encourage diving or jumping into shallow water.

- Don't use a tape deck around the pool that plugs into an electrical outlet. Instead, use battery-powered equipment.
- Don't teach exercises from the pool deck without using a mat or wearing appropriate foot gear.

If all the safety information in this chapter is applied in the class setting, participants will be safer and will feel that you care about them. They will be more apt to be comfortable with and committed to your instruction. In the next chapter we'll get to the actual lesson plans for your water exercise class. Instructions are given for teaching beginning, intermediate, and advanced level classes.

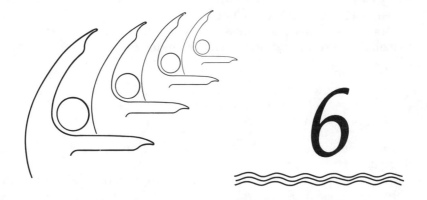

The Water Exercise Program Lesson Plans

The Y's Way to Water Exercise program is designed to accommodate a wide variety of ages and fitness levels in a single class. Some YMCAs may also offer classes that target special groups, such as athletes, pregnant women, people over 65, or those with arthritis. This chapter deals with only the more general approach to water exercise because this is most likely to be the type of class your YMCA offers. Formats for three levels of instruction are presented: beginning, intermediate, and advanced.

Class Design

Every class follows a standard overall format regardless of its level. The workout is structured to include exercise periods to develop all the components of physical fitness and warm-up and cool-down periods to help prevent injury. The format includes the following phases:

1. Warm-up
2. Aerobic exercises
3. Body exercises for flexibility, strength, and endurance
4. Cool-down

The three instructional levels vary in the time allocated to each of these phases, the number of exercises offered, and the intensity at which the exercises are conducted. (Remember to periodically increase the intensity of the exercises as the general fitness level of the class increases.)

The following is a review of the major concepts in each of the four phases of the session format.

Warm-Up   10-12 min.

> Rationale: —To raise the body's core temperature and adapt the body to the water's cooler temperature
> —To limber up the muscles
> —To increase muscle blood flow
> —To prepare the student mentally and emotionally for the more strenuous portion of the workout

- Warm up with both aerobic and stretching exercises.
- Emphasize static stretching rather than bouncing or ballistic stretching. Static stretching minimizes pain and strain to muscles.
- Use slow, rhythmic music to create a relaxed atmosphere and to encourage slow, steady movement.
- Have students move joints through their full range of motion.

Aerobic Exercises   15-20 min

> Rationale: —To improve the aerobic capacity of the heart and lungs by exercising the large muscle groups

- Use the program's aerobic exercises.
- Raise the heart rate to within the training heart rate range, usually between 65 and 85 percent of maximum heart rate. See Appendix F for the intensity rating of each aerobic exercise in the program.
- Maintain the heart rate within the training heart rate range during the aerobic phase so the cardiorespiratory system can adapt to the overload.
- Vary the angle of work for each muscle group frequently.
- Vary duration, frequency, and intensity to produce progressive overload as needed.
- Occasionally use swimmer's hand paddles to increase the intensity.

Body Exercises 10-15min

> Rationale: —To improve flexibility, muscular strength, and muscular endurance and to prevent muscle imbalance

- Use the exercises that focus on the upper, middle, and lower body.
- Improve students' flexibility by having them work the joints through their full range of motion and do static stretching.
- Develop students' muscle strength and tone by having them increase the force they use against the water's resistance during exercise. The muscles used for stabilizing the body during the exercise are also strengthened isometrically.
- Choose exercises to vary the angle of work for each muscle group.
- Occassionally use swimmer's hand paddles and kickboards to increase the intensity.

Cool-Down 10min

> Rationale: —To allow the heart rate to slow down and to stimulate continued blood flow
> —To prevent tightening or cramping of the muscles
> —To stop the pooling of blood in the lower extremities, thus preventing the build up of lactic acid. This helps prevent dizziness and nausea.

- Use exercises that stretch (static) the large muscle groups.
- Walking in the water should be used to allow for heart rate recovery.

- Cool down to relax and calm participants. This encourages their feeling good about the workout.

The Y's water exercise program is 8 weeks long, with three class meetings per week. Each class is based on a 1-hour session, but this may be adjusted according to your local Y's program schedule.

When water games or circuit-training activities are suggested, they should be conducted as part of the aerobic phase of the workout. You need to determine the time allotment for these special activities, keeping in mind that when combined with a portion of the regular aerobic workout, the total aerobic phase should still be 30 minutes long.

The three levels of instruction correspond to the three exercise levels described in *Y's Way to Water Exercise*. Level C is for beginners; Level B is for intermediate participants; and Level A is for advanced participants.

Beginning Level (Level C)

The essential thing to remember in teaching at this level is to start slowly and to emphasize correct performance in each exercise. Intensity in the first five to six classes is underplayed because more attention is given to basic performance instruction. Each student automatically selects a comfortable aerobic exercise pace, although he or she should attempt to reach a training heart rate level of 60 percent of maximum heart rate. General background music for atmosphere may be introduced in the fourth or fifth class, when the students appear to understand and perform the majority of the exercises properly. In the sixth or seventh class, music intended to regulate the rhythm (intensity) of exercise may be introduced.

Remember, beginning students experience different responses to exercise and are learning about themselves. You should go slowly and be supportive. Certain students may require special attention due to health problems or other physical limitations. Be understanding and help these individuals adapt to the exercises. Staying after class to counsel students with special problems is often very helpful. Once an adjustment is made, you will notice how such people tend to function well along with the rest of the class.

Lesson plans for a beginning course follow. Consult *Y's Way to Water Exercise*, Part II, "The Water Exercises." You should also refer to Appendix B, "List of Water Exercises," in the participant's text (p. 207) for a summary of all the exercises.

Here are the approximate amounts of time to be spent on the phases of the beginning-level workout. Note that the aerobic phase of the workout is gradually lengthened from 12 to 22 minutes as the participants' fitness levels improve.

Workout phase	Duration at start of course (minutes)	Duration at end of course (minutes)
Warm-up	5	5
Aerobics	12	22
Body exercises	18	18
Cool-down	5	5
Workout total	40	50

Beginning Level—Week 1

Class 1

- Fill out forms.
- Offer *Y's Way to Water Exercise* text.
- Present Minilecture 1, "Orientation to Water Exercise" (Appendix A).
- Show pool and discuss procedures, towels, lockers, and so on.
- Review exercise precautions (chapter 5, "Safety Concerns"), including danger signs during exercise.

Class 2

- Conduct the pretest. This can be the Y's Way to Physical Fitness test battery or the self-test in the participant's text (Appendix A, p. 205).
- Give Minilecture 2, "Use of Heart Rates in Exercise" (Appendix A).
- Calculate and record training heart rate ranges of 65 to 85 percent of maximum heart rate (participant's text, chapter 5, p. 47, and Appendix A, p. 206). Beginning participants should exercise at the 65 percent level at first.
- Teach how to take heart rates.
- Conduct a short workout as follows:

1
WARM-UP
Heel Slap (3)
Jumping Jacks (3)
Universal
Hip Dip

2
AEROBICS
Jumping Jacks (3)
Gerbil Wheel (2)
Heel Slap (3)
Bunny Hop (2)

3
BODY EXERCISES
Upper: Arm Circles
        Double Arm Lift and
          Press
Middle: Leap Frog
        Windshield Wiper
Lower: Leg Circles
        Pendulum

4
COOL-DOWN
Walk in chest-deep water.

Aerobic exercises are followed by numbers that indicate their intensity ratings (as shown in Appendix F).

Class 3

- Review workout phases: warm-up, aerobic exercises, body exercises, and cool-down.
- Teach the stabilizing positions (participant's text, pp. 60-62).
- Introduce good breathing technique.
- Correct improper exercise techniques or exercise intensity.
- Conduct the following workout and teach new exercises (shown in italics):

1
WARM-UP

Jumping Jacks (3)
Cross-Country Skier (2)
Hip Dip
Universal

2
AEROBICS

Heel Slap (3)
Downhiller (2)
Cossack Shuffle (1)
Bunny Hop (2)
Side Leg Side (2)
Joggernaut (1)

3
BODY EXERCISES

Upper: *Mae West*
       Wing Flap
       Arm Circles
       Shoulder Shrug
Middle: *Body Twist*
       Windshield Wiper
       Double Leg Lifts
Lower: Pendulum
       Lateral Lift
       Flamingo
       Ankle Action

4
COOL-DOWN

Heel Slap (very slow pace)
Chorus Line (very slow
   pace)
Walk in waist-deep water
for 2 minutes.

Beginning Level—Week 2

Class 4

- Conduct special demonstration on exercise intensity (chapter 4).
- Conduct the following workout and teach new exercises:

1
WARM-UP
Charleston Flap (3)
Jumping Jacks (3)
Hip Dip
Figurehead
Universal

2
AEROBICS
Bunny Hop (2)
Charleston Flap (3)
Charleston (2)
Gerbil Wheel (2)
One Leg Hop (3)
Scissors Jump (1)

3
BODY EXERCISES
Upper: *Figure 8*
    Agitator
    Arm Pendulum
Middle: *Fire Hydrant*
    Hula Hoop
Lower: *Half Moon*
    Plié
    Scissors Cross
    Wide Leg Kick

4
COOL-DOWN
Heel Slap (slow pace)
Joggernaut (slow pace)
Walk in waist-deep
    water for 1 minute.

- Introduce background music.
- Emphasize correct form.
- Take heart rates immediately after aerobic phase.

Class 5

- Repeat the workout from Class 4.
- Emphasize correct form and proper breathing.
- In this session, take heart rates at 2 minutes, 8 minutes, and at the end of the aerobic phase. Have participants check whether they are reaching their training heart rate ranges early in the workout.
- Give Minilecture 3, "Facts on Losing Weight" (Appendix A).

Class 6

- Revise the workout format as follows (note that the aerobic phase has been lengthened to 15 minutes):

1
WARM-UP
(5 minutes)

Select any 2 aerobic
 exercises, plus
Hip Dip
Figurehead
Universal

2
AEROBICS
(15 minutes)

Select any 10 exer-
 cises previously taught.

3
BODY EXERCISES
(18 minutes)

Select any 4 exercises
 from each category
 from exercises previ-
 ously taught.

4
COOL-DOWN
(5 minutes)

Walk in waist-deep
 water for 2 minutes.
Stretch out with the
 Universal and Hip
 Dip.

- Use music to control the rhythm (intensity) of the aerobic exercises.
- Take the heart rate as in Class 5.
- Emphasize getting a total workout and do less instruction.
- Stress the importance of being aware of the danger signs of exercise.
- Remember to vary the work angle of the aerobic exercises.

Beginning Level—Week 3

Class 7

- Continue to use the workout format from Class 6. Vary the selection of exercises.

1
WARM-UP
(5 minutes)

Select any 2 aerobic
exercises, plus
Hip Dip
Figurehead
Universal

2
AEROBICS
(15 minutes)

Select any 10 exercises previously taught.

3
BODY EXERCISES
(18 minutes)

Select any 4 exercises
from each category
from exercises previously taught.

4
COOL-DOWN
(5 minutes)

Walk in waist-deep water
for 2 minutes.
Stretch out with the
Universal and Hip Dip.

- Emphasize fun and socialization; permit light conversation.
- Increase the exercise intensity modestly.
- Inform students that stabilizing positions are also a form of isometric exercise—technique is important.
- Give Minilecture 4, "How to Maintain Your Exercise Program" (Appendix A).

Class 8

- Repeat the workout format from Class 6; continue to vary the selection of exercises.
- Concentrate on setting the pace for the exercise routine with the proper cadence or music beat.
- Stress landing on heels in aerobic exercises.

Class 9

- Repeat the workout format from Class 6, but reduce the total workout time to 30 minutes.
- Teach the following new aerobic exercises:
  Cheerleader Jump (1)
  Flutter Kick (1)
  High Jump (2)
  Polaris (2)
- Introduce the relaxation techniques from chapter 4.
- Give Minilecture 5, "Personalizing Your Program" (Appendix A).

Beginning Level—Week 4

Class 10

- Repeat the workout format from Class 6.

1
WARM-UP
(5 minutes)

Select any 2 aerobic
exercises, plus
Hip Dip
Figurehead
Universal

2
AEROBICS
(15 minutes)

Select any 10 exercises
previously taught.

3
BODY EXERCISES
(18 minutes)

Select any 4 exercises from
each category from exer-
cises previously taught.

4
COOL-DOWN
(5 minutes)

Walk in waist-deep water for
2 minutes.
Stretch out with the Universal
and Hip Dip.

- Teach the following upper body exercises and add 2 previously
  taught exercises for a total of 4 in this group:
  Golf Swing
  Quack, Quack
- Teach the following lower body exercises and add 2 previously
  taught exercises for a total of 4 in this group:
  Left Right Left
  Swift Kick

Class 11

- Repeat the workout format from Class 6 and continue to vary the
  selection of exercises.
- Teach the following middle body exercises and add 2 previously
  taught exercises for a total of 4 in this group:
  Modified Scissors Cross
  Six Count Twister

Class 12

- Revise the workout format as follows (note that the aerobic phase has been lengthened to 18 minutes):

1
WARM-UP
(5 minutes)
Select any 2 aerobic
  exercises, plus
Hip Dip
Figurehead
Universal

2
AEROBICS
(18 minutes)
Select any 12 exercises
  previously taught.

3
BODY EXERCISES
(18 minutes)
Select any 4 exercises from
  each category from exercises previously taught.

4
COOL-DOWN
(5 minutes)
Walk in waist-deep water for
  3 minutes.
Stretch out with the Universal and Hip Dip.

- In the aerobics phase, begin to alternate the exercises with respect to their angles of movement (e.g., Side Leg Side, lateral; Charleston, oblique; Cossack Shuffle, frontal). Do not use more than 2 exercises at any one angle because the muscles may begin to fatigue.

Beginning Level—Week 5

Class 13

- Continue with the workout format from Class 12.

1
WARM-UP
(5 minutes)
Select any 2 aerobic
exercises, plus
Hip Dip
Figurehead
Universal

2
AEROBICS
(18 minutes)
Select any 12 exercises
previously taught.

3
BODY EXERCISES
(18 minutes)
Select any 4 exercises from
each category from exer-
cises previously taught.

4
COOL-DOWN
(5 minutes)
Walk in waist-deep water
for 3 minutes.
Stretch out with the
Universal and Hip Dip.

- Teach the following upper body exercises for a total of 4 for this
category:
Shake
Tidal Wave
Traffic Cop
Wrist Action
- Use the relaxation techniques suggested in chapter 4.

Class 14

- Conduct a 30-minute workout as in Class 9.
- Allow 15 minutes for introducing a water game (Appendix C).
- Give Minilecture 6, "Everyone Can Perform Water Exercise" (Ap-
pendix A).

Class 15

- Continue with the format from Class 12.
- Teach the following lower body exercises:
Leg Stretch
Quad Stretch
Calf Builder

Beginning Level—Week 6

Classes 16 and 17

- Repeat the workout format from Class 12.

1
WARM-UP
(5 minutes)
Select any 2 aerobic
exercises, plus
Hip Dip
Figurehead
Universal

2
AEROBICS
(18 minutes)
Select any 12 exercises
previously taught.

3
BODY EXERCISES
(18 minutes)
Select any 4 exercises from
each category from exer-
cises previously taught.

4
COOL-DOWN
(5 minutes)
Walk in waist-deep water for
3 minutes.
Stretch out with the Universal
and Hip Dip.

- Use games occasionally.
- Increase the exercise intensity to the 70 percent maximum heart rate level.
- Give Minilecture 7, "Injuries and Water Exercise" (Appendix A), in Class 17.

Class 18

- Revise the workout format as follows (note that the aerobic phase has been lengthened to 22 minutes):

1
WARM-UP
(5 minutes)
Select any 3 aerobic
exercises, plus
Universal
Hip Dip
Figurehead

3
BODY EXERCISES
(18 minutes)
Select any 5 exercises from
each category.

(Continued)

2
AEROBICS
(22 minutes)
Select any 16 exercises.

4
COOL-DOWN
(5 minutes)
Select any 3 aerobic exercises and perform them at a slow cadence.

• Emphasize attaining training heart rates.

Beginning Level—Week 7

Classes 19, 20, and 21

- Repeat the workout format from Class 18.

1
WARM-UP
(5 minutes)

Select any 3 aerobic
exercises, plus
Universal
Hip Dip
Figurehead

2
AEROBICS
(22 minutes)

Select any 16 exercises.

3
BODY EXERCISES
(18 minutes)

Select any 5 exercises from
each category.

4
COOL-DOWN
(5 minutes)

Select any 3 aerobic exercises and perform them at
a slow cadence.

- In Class 20 substitute a circuit-training program for the entire class. (See chapter 4 and Appendix B for a discussion of circuit training.)
- Increase exercise intensity to the 75 percent maximum heart rate level.
- Give Minilecture 8, "Your Results From Exercise" (Appendix A), in Class 21.

Beginning Level—Week 8

Class 22

- Repeat the workout format from Class 18.

Class 23

- Begin posttesting.
- Conduct a short aerobic workout if time permits.

Class 24

- Finish posttesting.
- Play water games if time permits.
- Give a farewell speech and encourage participants to register for the intermediate class.
- Present awards, certificates, T-shirts, and so on.

Intermediate Level (Level B)

The intermediate-level class is designed for participants who have at least average fitness. Therefore, it is important that everyone who signs up for this course be properly screened. A person should be allowed to register for an intermediate course only if he or she has met at least one of the two following conditions:

- Has participated in the beginning class and can perform aerobic exercises at a training heart rate of 70 to 75 percent of maximum heart rate. Anyone who has completed a beginning class but has not improved to the 70 to 75 percent level should be asked to *repeat* the beginning class.
- Has taken the intermediate course but has let too much time elapse to go on to the advanced class. This person should be able to perform aerobic exercises at a training heart rate of 70 to 75 percent of maximum heart rate.

The participant's goal for the intermediate course should be to improve the training heart rate to the 75 to 80 percent level. If the students do not consistently improve their training heart rates and/or do not have the enthusiasm to reach an advanced level of fitness, it may be necessary to conduct the class with the aim of *maintaining* average fitness levels (75 percent of maximum heart rate).

These are the approximate amounts of time to be spent on each phase of the intermediate-level workout:

Workout phase	Duration at start of course (minutes)	Duration at end of course (minutes)
Warm-up	5	5
Aerobics	20	30
Body exercises	20	20
Cool-down	5	5
Workout Total	50	60

Intermediate Level—Week 1

Class 1

- Fill out forms.
- Review physical fitness concepts in Minilecture 1 from beginner's class.
- Review exercise precautions, including danger signs during exercise (chapter 5).
- Conduct a short workout emphasizing aerobics (follow the same aerobic workout as in Class 3 of the beginner's level, but at a greater intensity).

Class 2

- Pretest if previous test was taken more than 4 weeks ago.
- Emphasize exercise intensity (chapter 4).
- Calculate and record training heart rate ranges of 65 to 85 percent of maximum heart rate (participants' text, chapter 5, p. 47, and Appendix A, p. 206). Intermediate participants should exercise at the 70 percent level at first.
- Stress the importance of checking heart rate after each aerobic workout.
- Conduct a complete but reduced workout as in Class 3 of the beginner's level, reviewing and emphasizing body exercises.

Class 3

- Begin a regular workout using the following exercises in order:

1
WARM-UP

Jumping Jacks (3)
Downhiller (2)
Universal
Hip Dip
Figurehead

2
AEROBICS

Heel Slap (3)
Gerbil Wheel (2)
Cross-Country Skier (2)

3
BODY EXERCISES

Upper: Shoulder Shrug
Golf Swing
Arm Circles
Mae West
Wing Flap
Middle: Leap Frog
Six Count Twister
Windshield Wiper
Double Leg Lift
Fire Hydrant
Lower: Flamingo
Pendulum

2
AEROBICS

Charleston (2)
Joggernaut (1)
Jumping Jacks (3)
Polaris (2)
Cossack Shuffle (1)
Scissors Jump (1)

3
BODY EXERCISES

Lower: Lateral Lifts
       Left Right Left
       Calf Builder

4
COOL-DOWN

Walk slowly for 3 minutes.
Do the Heel Slap slowly.

• Remember to vary the work angle in the aerobic exercises.

Aerobic exercises are followed by numbers that indicate their intensity ratings (as shown in Appendix F).

Intermediate Level—Week 2

Class 4

- Review exercise precautions (chapter 5, "Safety Concerns").
- Continue with a regular workout, using the following exercise format:

1
WARM-UP

Heel Slap (3)
One Leg Hop (3)
Hip Dip
Universal
Figurehead

2
AEROBICS

Jumping Jacks (3)
Polaris (2)
Side Leg Side (2)
Cossack Shuffle (1)
Cheerleader Jump (1)
Bunny Hop (2)
Chorus Line (3)
High Jump (2)
Flutter Kick (1)
Downhiller (2)
Charleston Flap (3)

3
BODY EXERCISES

Upper: Shake
        Mae West
        Tidal Wave
        Wrist Action
        Arm Pendulum
        Double Arm Lift
          and Press
Middle: Double Leg Lift
        Fire Hydrant
        Six Count Twister
        Leap Frog
Lower: Leg Circles
        Ankle Action
        Plié
        Half Moon
        Scissors Cross
        Leg Stretch

4
COOL-DOWN

Walk slowly for 3 minutes.
Do the Downhiller slowly.

- Emphasize good exercise form and technique.
- Introduce background music.

Class 5

- Use music for aerobic rhythm.
- Continue with a regular workout using the following exercise format:

1
WARM-UP
Joggernaut (1)
High Jump (2)
Universal
Hip Dip
Six Count Twister

2
AEROBICS
Downhiller (2)
One Leg Hop (3)
Cheerleader Jump (1)
Cossack Shuffle (1)
Joggernaut (1)
Charleston (2)
High Jump (2)
Scissors Jump (1)
Flutter Kick (1)
Side Leg Side (2)
Cheerleader Jump (1)

3
BODY EXERCISES
Upper: Agitator
Figure 8
Quack, Quack
Traffic Cop
Middle: Body Twist
Hip Dip
Modified Scissors
Cross
Six Count Twister
Leap Frog
Fire Hydrant
Lower: Pendulum
Lateral Lifts
Quad Stretch
Swift Kick
Wide Leg Kick
Flamingo
Leg Circles

4
COOL-DOWN
Do the Joggernaut slowly
for 3 minutes.
Walk slowly.

• Use moderately paced music.

Class 6
• Repeat the workout from Class 3.
• Use faster-paced choreographed music.
• Review exercise intensity (chapter 4).

Intermediate Level—Week 3

Class 7

- Repeat the workout format from Class 5.

1
WARM-UP
Joggernaut (1)
High Jump (2)
Universal
Hip Dip
Six Count Twister

2
AEROBICS
Downhiller (2)
One Leg Hop (3)
Cheerleader Jump (1)
Cossack Shuffle (1)
Joggernaut (1)
Charleston (2)
High Jump (2)
Scissors Jump (1)
Flutter Kick (1)
Side Leg Side (2)
Cheerleader Jump (1)

3
BODY EXERCISES
Upper: Agitator
 Figure 8
 Quack, Quack
 Traffic Cop
Middle: Body Twist
 Hip Dip
 Modified Scissors
 Cross
 Six Count Twister
 Leap Frog
 Fire Hydrant
Lower: Pendulum
 Lateral Lift
 Quad Stretch
 Swift Kick
 Wide Leg Kick
 Flamingo
 Leg Circles

4

COOL-DOWN
Do the Joggernaut slowly
 for 3 minutes.
Walk slowly.

- Use body exercises from Class 5 but rearrange the order in each group.
- Give Minilecture 1, "Motivation" (Appendix A).

Class 8

- Repeat the workout format from Class 4.

1
WARM-UP

Heel Slap (3)
One Leg Hop (3)
Hip Dip
Universal
Figurehead

2
AEROBICS

Jumping Jacks (3)
Polaris (2)
Side Leg Side (2)
Cossack Shuffle (1)
Cheerleader Jump (1)
Bunny Hop (2)
Chorus Line (3)
High Jump (2)
Flutter Kick (1)
Downhiller (2)
Charleston Flap (3)

3
BODY EXERCISES

Upper: Shake
Mae West
Tidal Wave
Wrist Action
Arm Pendulum
Double Arm Lift
and Press
Middle: Double Leg Lift
Fire Hydrant
Six Count Twister
Leap Frog
Lower: Leg Circles
Ankle Action
Plié
Half Moon
Scissors Cross
Leg Stretch

4
COOL-DOWN

Walk slowly for 3 minutes.
Do the Downhiller slowly.

- In the aerobic phase, teach the exercises in groups based on intensity levels. Use the following sequence: 3s, 2s; then 1s. (See Appendix F for intensity levels of aerobic exercises.)
- Use faster-paced music.

Class 9

- Repeat the workout format from Class 5.
- Vary the aerobic exercises used in the warm-up.
- In the aerobic phase, teach the exercises in groups based on intensity levels.
- Use the following sequence: 3s, 2s, then 1s. Increase the pace of the 2s.

Intermediate Level—Week 4

Classes 10 and 11

• Repeat the workout format from Class 4.

1
WARM-UP

Heel Slap (3)
One Leg Hop (3)
Hip Dip
Universal
Figurehead

2
AEROBICS

Jumping Jacks (3)
Polaris (2)
Side Leg Side (2)
Cossack Shuffle (1)
Cheerleader Jump (1)
Bunny Hop (2)
Chorus Line (3)
High Jump (2)
Flutter Kick (1)
Downhiller (2)
Charleston Flap (3)

3
BODY EXERCISES

Upper: Shake
       Mae West
       Tidal Wave
       Wrist Action
       Arm Pendulum
       Double Arm Lift
         and Press
Middle: Double Leg Lift
        Fire Hydrant
        Six Count Twister
        Leap Frog
Lower: Leg Circles
       Ankle Action
       Plié
       Half Moon
       Scissors Cross
       Leg Stretch

4
COOL-DOWN

Walk slowly for 3 minutes.
Do the Downhiller slowly.

• In the aerobic phase, introduce circuit training for at least one class session as follows (See chapter 4, "Teaching Methodology"):

Station 1	Charleston Flap (3)
Station 2	Downhiller (2)
Station 3	One Leg Hop (3)
Station 4	Cossack Shuffle (1)
Station 5	Chorus Line (3)
Station 6	Polaris (2)
Station 7	Joggernaut (1)

Station 8   Scissors Jump (1)
Station 9   Cheerleader Jump (1)
Station 10   High Jump (2)

Class 12

- Continue the workouts with the following exercise format (note that the aerobic phase has been lengthened to 25 minutes):

1
WARM-UP
(5 minutes)

Select any 2 aerobic
  exercises, plus
Hip Dip
Figurehead
Universal

2
AEROBICS
(25 minutes)

Select any 12 exercises.

3
BODY EXERCISES
(20 minutes)

Select any 5 exercises from
  each category.

4
COOL-DOWN
(5 minutes)

Do the Joggernaut slowly
  for 2 minutes.
Walk slowly.

Intermediate Level—Week 5

Class 13

- Repeat the workout format from Class 12.

1
WARM-UP
(5 minutes)

Select any 2 aerobic
exercises, plus
Hip Dip
Figurehead
Universal

2
AEROBICS
(25 minutes)

Select any 12 exercises.

3
BODY EXERCISES
(20 minutes)

Select any 5 exercises from
each category.

4
COOL-DOWN
(5 minutes)

Do the Joggernaut slowly
for 2 minutes.
Walk slowly.

- Use the circuit-training method from Classes 10 and 11 for the aerobic phase.
- Vary the selection of body exercises.
- Introduce relaxation techniques and use them when time permits in all subsequent workouts (chapter 4).

Class 14

- Repeat the workout format from Class 12.
- Vary the order in which you teach the aerobic exercises.
- Begin to increase the pace of the exercises rated 2s and 3s.
- Vary the selection of body exercises.
- Give Minilecture 2, "Nutrition" (Appendix A).

Class 15

- Repeat the workout format from Class 12.
- Use hand paddles during the aerobic workout to increase resistance.
- Vary the selection of body exercises.
- Reemphasize the importance of taking training heart rates.

Intermediate Level—Week 6

Class 16

- Repeat the workout format from Class 12.

1
WARM-UP
(5 minutes)
Select any 2 aerobic
exercises, plus
Hip Dip
Figurehead
Universal

2
AEROBICS
(25 minutes)
Select any 12 exercises.

3
BODY EXERCISES
(20 minutes)
Select any 5 exercises from
each category.

4
COOL-DOWN
(5 minutes)
Do the Joggernaut slowly
for 2 minutes.
Walk slowly.

- Organize all 12 aerobic exercises into 3 groups according to the following intensity-rating sequence: 2s (1 exercise), 1s (2 exercises), 3s (1 exercise). Perform each group once.
- Vary the selection of body exercises.
- Increase exercise intensity to the 80 percent maximum heart rate level.

Class 17

- Repeat the workout format from Class 16.
- Add a fourth group for a total of 16 aerobic exercises and lengthen this phase to *30* minutes.
- In the body exercise phase, perform 6 middle body exercises 2 minutes each (12 minutes), but only 4 upper and 4 lower body exercises 1 minute each (8 minutes).

Class 18

- Repeat the workout format from Class 17.
- Use circuit training for the aerobic phase (refer to Classes 10 and 11 but change a few of the exercises). Vary the time spent on each exercise, emphasizing the high-intensity exercises.
- Decrease the time spent in the body exercises phase to allow for Minilecture 3, "Aging and Exercise" (Appendix A).

Intermediate Level—Week 7

Classes 19, 20, and 21

- Continue the format from Class 17 for each of the workouts this week.
- Occasionally use hand paddles in the aerobic phase.
- Introduce hand paddles and/or kickboards in the following upper body exercises: Arm Pendulum, Double Arm Lift and Press, Golf Swing, and Wing Flap. Have participants hold kickboards in outstretched arms.

Intermediate Level—Week 8

Class 22

- Select any workout format from a previous class.
- Use water games for the aerobic phase.

Class 23

- Start posttesting.
- Conduct a short aerobic workout if time permits.

Class 24

- Finish posttesting.
- Play water games if time permits.
- Give awards and farewell speech.
- Encourage participants to register for the advanced class.

Advanced Level (Level A)

This course is intended for serious physical fitness enthusiasts and athletes who realize the advantages of exercising in the water. You might encourage people who are actively engaged in other forms of physical activity and athletics to consider adding a partial workout in the water. For this reason, it may be to your Y's advantage to set aside two or three advanced classes and promote them as an "open" or "introductory-offer" type of class to the Y membership. These sessions might include minilectures on how water exercise may help improve athletic performance or be used in injury rehabilitation.

A person should be allowed to register for an advanced course only if he or she has the ability to perform at a training heart rate of 75 percent of maximum heart rate. While previous participation in a water exercise class is preferred, it is not necessary.

The main goal of the advanced class is to produce a high-level aerobic workout, challenging the participants at the 85 percent of maximum heart rate level. You should emphasize obtaining maximum levels of flexibility, strength, and muscular endurance.

Following are the approximate durations of the phases of the advanced-level workout:

Workout phase	*Duration (minutes)*
Warm-up	5
Aerobics	30
Body exercises	20
Cool-down	5
Workout total	60

Advanced Level—Week 1

Class 1

- Fill out forms.
- Review physical fitness concepts and discuss the importance of a total-fitness approach to exercise (participant's text, chapter 1; instructor's guide, chapter 3).
- Review exercise precautions, including danger signs during exercise (chapter 5).
- Conduct a short workout emphasizing aerobic exercises; choose 6 aerobic exercises and 2 body exercises from each category.

Class 2

- Pretest if previous test was taken more than 4 weeks ago.
- Calculate and record training heart rate ranges of 65 to 85 percent of maximum heart rate (participant's text, chapter 5, p. 47, and Appendix A, p. 206). Advanced participants should exercise at the 75 percent level or above at first.
- Stress the importance of checking heart rate after each aerobic workout.
- Conduct a short workout emphasizing the body exercises; choose 5 aerobic exercises and 3 body exercises from each category.

Class 3

- Conduct a regular workout using the following exercise format (teach the exercises in the order presented):

1
WARM-UP

One Leg Hop (3)
Side Leg Side (2)
Figurehead
Universal
Hip Dip

2
AEROBICS

Heel Slap (3)
Gerbil Wheel (2)
Cheerleader Jump (1)
Charleston (2)

3
BODY EXERCISES

Upper: Mae West
Arm Circles
Wing Flap
Figure 8
Agitator
Middle: Double Leg Lift
Modified Scissors
Cross
Body Twist
Hula Hoop
Windshield Wiper
Lower: Calf Builder
Ankle Action

(Continued)

2
AEROBICS

Joggernaut (1)
Side Leg Side (2)
Flutter Kick (1)
Cross-Country Skier (2)
High Jump (2)

3
BODY EXERCISES

Lower: Left Right Left
        Pendulum
        Scissors Cross

4
COOL-DOWN

Do the Joggernaut for 3
  minutes.
Walk slowly.

• Use moderately paced music.

Aerobic exercises are followed by numbers that indicate their intensity ratings (as shown in Appendix F).

Advanced Level—Week 2

Class 4

- Continue with the following workout format:

1
WARM-UP

Select any 3 aerobic
  exercises, plus
Hip Dip
Figurehead
Universal

2
AEROBICS

Select any 14 aerobic
  exercises.

3
BODY EXERCISES

Select any 5 exercises from
  each category.

4
COOL-DOWN

Select an aerobic exercise;
  perform it at a slow pace
  for 2 minutes.
Walk slowly.

- Select exercises from the aerobic group (participant's text, Appendix B, p. 207)
- Remember to vary the aerobic exercises according to their angle of work. (See Appendix F for angle of work of each exercise.)

Classes 5 and 6

- Repeat the workout format from Class 4.
- Rearrange the aerobic exercises into groups based upon intensity levels; teach all 3s, then the 2s, then the 1s (see Appendix F for intensity levels of aerobics exercises).
- Use moderately paced music.
- In Class 6 give Minilecture 1, "Sports Performance" (Appendix A).

Advanced Level—Week 3

Class 7

- Repeat the workout format from Class 4.

1
WARM-UP

Select any 3 aerobic
  exercises, plus
Hip Dip
Figurehead
Universal

2
AEROBICS

Select any 14 aerobic
  exercises.

3
BODY EXERCISES

Select any 5 exercises from
  each category.

4
COOL-DOWN

Select an aerobic exercise;
  perform it at a slow pace
  for 2 minutes.
Walk slowly.

- Increase the intensity of the aerobic phase; begin to work at the
  80 percent of maximum heart rate level.

Class 8

- Repeat the workout format from Class 4.
- Use circuit training for the aerobic phase as follows:

Station 1	Joggernaut (1)
Station 2	High Jump (2)
Station 3	Cheerleader Jump (1)
Station 4	Flutter Kick (1)
Station 5	Heel Slap (3)
Station 6	Gerbil Wheel (2)
Station 7	Scissors Jump (1)
Station 8	Cossack Shuffle (1)
Station 9	Cross-Country Skier (2)
Station 10	Cheerleader Jump (1)

- Signal a change after 3 minutes at each station.
- Use moderately to fast paced music.

Class 9

- Repeat the workout format from Class 4.
- Select only aerobic exercises rated at an intensity of 1 or 2.
- Use faster music to increase the exercise intensity.
- Give Minilecture 2, "Injuries" (Appendix A).

Advanced Level—Week 4

Class 10

- Continue with the workout format from Class 4. Add one more exercise to the aerobic phase for a total of 15.

1
WARM-UP

Select any 3 aerobic
  exercises, plus
Hip Dip
Figurehead
Universal

2
AEROBICS

Select any 15 aerobic
  exercises.

3
BODY EXERCISES

Select any 5 exercises from
  each category.

4
COOL-DOWN

Select an aerobic exercise;
  perform it at a slow pace
  for 2 minutes.
Walk slowly.

- Use the relaxation techniques suggested in chapter 4 at the end of class and continue to use in subsequent classes when time permits.

Class 11

- Repeat the workout format from Class 10.
- Organize all 15 aerobic exercises into groups of 3 according to the following intensity-rating sequence: two 1s followed by a 2. Perform each group once.
- Use fast music.
- Give Minilecture 3, "Advanced Fitness" (Appendix A).

Class 12

- Repeat the workout format from Class 10.
- Begin to increase the aerobic intensity to the 85 percent of maximum heart rate level.
- Add hand paddles to the aerobic phase, but tell students to discontinue their use if the workout becomes too difficult or pain is experienced.
- Perform the body exercise phase with the following exercise sequence:

Upper: Arm Pendulum
        Quack, Quack
        Shoulder Shrug
        Tidal Wave
        Traffic Cop

Middle: Fire Hydrant
        Hip Dip
        Six Count Twister
        Double Leg Lift
        Hula Hoop

Lower: Flamingo
        Leg Circles
        Plié
        Swift Kick
        Quad Stretch

Advanced Level—Week 5

Classes 13, 14, and 15

- Repeat the workout format from Class 10.

1
WARM-UP

Select any 3 aerobic
  exercises, plus
Hip Dip
Figurehead
Universal

2
AEROBICS

Select any 15 aerobic
  exercises.

3
BODY EXERCISES

Select any 5 exercises from
  each category.

4
COOL-DOWN

Select an aerobic exercise;
  perform it at a slow pace
  for 2 minutes.
Walk slowly.

- Vary the aerobic phase as follows:

  a. Use circuit training as in Class 8 but substitute at least 5 different aerobic exercises (your choice) for a total of 10 exercise stations.

  b. Play Inner Tube Water Polo or conduct Water Relay Races (see Appendix C).

- Continue with moderately to fast paced music (no more than 3 exercises at the same angle).

Advanced Level—Week 6

Classes 16, 17, 18

- Use the following workout format:

1
WARM-UP

Let the class choose 3 of their favorite aerobic exercises and 4 stretching exercises.

2
AEROBICS

Have students perform the following exercises in a circular pattern of movement for a total of 9 minutes: Joggernaut, Bunny Hop, High Jump, and Polaris. Give commands to periodically change direction. Then select 7 exercises and perform them for 3 minutes each.

3
BODY EXERCISES

Have students choose the first 3 exercises in each category and you choose 3 for a total of 18 exercises.

4
COOL-DOWN

Have the whole class perform the Gerbil Wheel in a circle slowly for 2 minutes and then walk slowly in any direction for 2 minutes. Stretch out with the Universal exercise.

- In Class 18 change the aerobic workout by organizing 15 aerobic exercises into groups of 5 according to the following intensity rating sequence: four 1s and a 2. Perform each group once. Allow 2 minutes for each exercise.
- Increase the exercise intensity to the 85 percent maximum heart rate level.

Advanced Level—Week 7

Classes 19, 20, 21

- Use the following workout format:

1
WARM-UP

Perform the Joggernaut and
   High Jump in a circular pat-
   tern, plus
Hip Dip
Universal

3
BODY EXERCISES

Select and perform 4 exercises in the upper and lower
   body category (1 ½ minutes
   each) and 8 middle body
   exercises (1 minute each)

2
AEROBICS

Let students select and perform their 12 favorite exercises for 2 ½ minutes each

4
COOL-DOWN

Have students select 2
   aerobic exercises and
   perform them slowly.
Walk slowly for 2 minutes.

- In Class 19, try to organize the 12 aerobic exercises into 3 groups
  of 4 according to the following intensity rating sequence: 1, 2,
  1, 2. Perform each group once. Try to vary the angles at which
  the muscles work as well.
- In Class 20, select 15 aerobic exercises. Choose ones with an intensity rating of 1 or 2 and vary the angles at which the muscles
  work.
- In Class 21, select 5 aerobic exercises rated 1 and 2 in intensity
  and perform 3 minutes each. Then use the class's favorite water
  games for the remaining 15 minutes (see Appendix C).

Advanced Level—Week 8

Class 22

- Conduct a warm-up using the students' favorite exercises.
- Organize the class into teams for water relay races during the remainder of the class (see Appendix C).

Class 23

- Start posttesting.
- Conduct a short aerobic workout if time permits.

Class 24

- Finish posttesting.
- Play water games if time permits.
- Distribute awards and give farewell speech.

The lesson plans provided here should give you what you need for teaching classes at the beginning, intermediate, and advanced levels. Because you may find that during the course of the lessons people may ask you questions about nutrition and weight management, the following chapter gives you some information on those topics.

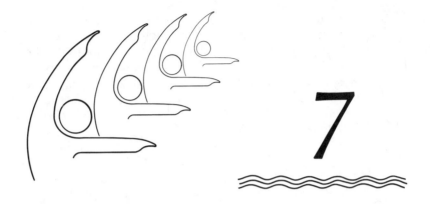

Nutrition and Weight Management Concepts

As an instructor teaching a physical fitness class, you need to teach your students some basic information about diet and exercise. This chapter provides enough information on nutrition and weight management for you to plan minilectures for your class. Additional information may be obtained by consulting the book *Y's Way to Weight Management* and chapter 11, "Weight Conscious: Applying the Magic Formula," in *Y's Way to Water Exercise*.

Nutrition

The foods we eat contain nutrients. Nutrients are chemical substances in food—made usable to the body by digestion, absorption, and bloodstream transport—that are necessary for such bodily functions as the production of energy for normal daily activity, the building and maintenance of body cells, and the regulation of a multitude of physiological processes. Nutrients in the food we eat are divided into six categories:

- Carbohydrates
- Protein
- Fat
- Minerals
- Vitamins
- Water

The combination and amounts of nutrients we consume are important and can have a serious impact on exercise and athletic performance. People who exercise regularly are mainly concerned with carbohydrates (sugars and starches), because they are the primary source of energy for muscle activity. Carbohydrates are digested more easily than fats or proteins and end up in the bloodstream as a simple chemical substance called *glucose*. Glucose that is not used for energy is converted into *glycogen* and stored in the muscles and liver for future energy needs. Once the glycogen stores are full, the excess glucose is converted into fat and stored in fat cells (adipose tissue).

Sports that require sustained efforts of approximately 30 minutes or more may eventually deplete athletes' glycogen stores. Athletes in these activities (distance runners, for example) who fail to replenish their bodies with carbohydrates will become fatigued, and their performances will suffer. Without adequate carbohydrate stores, the body turns to fat stores for energy and, after that, to protein, which is the least efficient source of energy.

Athletes who plan to engage in prolonged aerobic exercise sometimes resort to "carbohydrate loading" before their events. They eat foods rich in complex carbohydrates, such as pastas and whole grains, in order to build up their glycogen reserves.

Your students probably won't want to overload on carbohydrates, because most of them are not involved in high-level athletic training. However, it's good for everyone to know the value of nutrients, in order to choose a well-balanced diet or eating pattern. Protein is primarily used for muscle growth and maintenance. Vitamins, minerals, and water are important in the chemical reactions that release energy. In addition, *vitamins* help maintain normal cell operations. They are widely available in the foods we eat. Vitamin supplements are not usually needed if one eats a balanced diet. *Minerals* also play a supporting role in helping control bodily processes and affect the distribution of water within the body. Mineral supplements are also unnecessary if one eats a healthy diet. *Water* makes up 60 percent of body weight and has many functions: It aids in the elimination of wastes, assists in the digestive process, acts as a coolant in the body, makes up a portion of the blood, and acts as a lubricant in the internal organs and joints. Unfortunately, most people do not drink enough water. It is recommended that a person drink at least six to eight glasses of water every day.

The best advice to give to your students is that they should eat three meals a day, selecting a variety of food from the four major food groups: meats, dairy products, fruits and vegetables, and grains. The meat group includes various nonmeat protein sources, such as beans, nuts, and seeds.

Here is a simple list of guidelines for healthy eating:

1. *Eat a variety of foods.* No single food provides all the nutrients a person needs. Therefore, it is important to eat a variety of foods to ensure that you are getting all the essential nutrients.
2. *Avoid too much sugar.* Sugars are high in calories and low in vitamins and minerals. It is best to limit consumption of sugar as it is present in many processed foods that we eat.
3. *Avoid too much fat.* The main concern here is that although fat is the most concentrated source of energy, some fats, especially saturated ones, have been shown to be contributing factors in heart disease. Cholesterol, a fat-like substance found only in animal (and human) cells, also increases the risk for heart disease when found in high levels in the blood.
4. *Eat foods with ample starch and fiber.* Most Americans eat a diet that is too low in starch and fiber. A high-fiber diet can reduce the risk of colon and rectal cancer. Dietary starch and fiber can be increased by your eating fruits and vegetables, potatoes, whole grain breads and cereals, peas, and beans.
5. *Avoid too much sodium (salt).* Too much sodium in the diet can contribute to high blood pressure, especially with people who have a family history of high blood pressure. Left untreated, high blood pressure may lead to heart attacks, strokes, and kidney disease. A large amount of salt in the diet also causes the body to retain water.

6. *If you consume alcohol, do so in moderation.* Drinking too much alcohol has been associated with many health problems, such as cancers of the liver, mouth, and throat. If people smoke and drink, they compound their risk. Also, alcohol is high in calories and low in vitamins and minerals.

7. *Drink water.* Drink at least 6 to 8 glasses of water per day. Fluids like juices, electrolyte drinks, and so on are not substitutes for water, because they contain soluble material that causes the fluid to stay in the stomach longer during digestion. This fact is particularly pertinent for athletes who need to process water through the digestive system rapidly for the production of sweat and prevention of dehydration.

8. *Eat at regular times.* Eating at regular intervals throughout the day helps facilitate the digestive process. It also encourages regular bowel movements. Human beings are basically creatures of habit, and biological functions seem to be more efficient when a regular pattern of activity is established.

Challenge your students to review their eating habits. They will know where they are lacking. If they wish to eat healthy, they may have to modify their habits—and that means changing their lifestyles. It won't be easy, but with some encouragement from you, they will be able to make these changes.

Weight Management

Eating healthy also means not gaining excess weight. If you don't believe this, ask the students in your next class session how many of them are there in order to lose weight. Probably more than half of the students will raise their hands. Of all the reasons people exercise, losing weight seems to be one of the most popular.

Dieting and Exercise

Most of the students wanting to lose weight have probably tried a number of diet plans without much success. They eventually come to the realization that a successful weight-loss program depends on a combination of diet and *exercise*. They have learned that dieting by itself does not guarantee permanent weight loss.

When a person only diets, the weight that is lost is a combination of fat and muscle, the proportion sometimes as high as 50-50. This means that if 20 pounds were lost, 10 pounds would be fat and 10 pounds muscle. Problems begin when the weight is gained back: All the weight gain is probably fat, and too much fat is unhealthy.

Well, what is so important about muscle? For most people, having well-proportioned musculature with good muscle tone is appealing because it is visually attractive. The less fortunate, with their sagging muscles, look overweight and sedentary.

A more vital consideration is the quantity and efficiency of muscle and how well it performs during physical activity. In addition to its primary function of performing everyday tasks with adequate strength, muscle is essential in controlling weight because its activity burns large amounts of calories. This is easy to understand: Every muscle is made up of many muscle fibers, each of which may be viewed as a small power unit. During activity, digested food provides energy to working muscles. Large amounts of calories (a measure of the energy-releasing potential of food) can be used up this way, especially if large muscle groups are recruited in this activity. If the activity is aerobic and sustained for a long period of time (approximately 30 minutes), the body calls on the immediately available energy nutrients, carbohydrates, before it uses the stored fats for energy. It's after burning carbohydrates that a person can begin to lose unwanted, bulging fat.

Another reason that muscle is important—one that is often overlooked—is that while the body is at rest, the muscles are still burning calories to maintain basic biological functions. This is called *basal metabolism*. The more muscle on a body's frame, the more calories burned. This is a very significant factor and may be one of the best explanations why people need to exercise when they diet. *Exercise builds and improves muscle function, which in turn burns calories, even during rest, causing a person to lose fat weight, not muscle weight!*

Consider two individuals each weighing 150 pounds, with one (individual A) having more fat and less muscle than the other (individual B). Individual B is going to burn more calories at rest than A because of the greater muscle mass. When these two people exercise, B again is going to burn more calories.

A person who wants to lose weight from certain areas of the body needs to know that fat is lost according to one's genetic design. In addition, fat loss usually begins with the last place fat was stored. Those facts mean that some people may lose weight in the face first, the hips next, then the stomach, and so on. People often become discouraged when it takes too long for weight to be lost from certain locations. They need to be told not to give up, because they will *eventually* lose weight from where they desire. Plenty of aerobic exercise will help them reach their goal.

Calorie Consciousness

The "magic formula" for losing weight simply states that an individual needs to decrease caloric intake and increase caloric expenditure. This means that in addition to fewer calories' being consumed (and this may mean smaller quantities of food), physical activity needs to be increased.

To be calorie-conscious means to be weight-conscious, which is a term preferred to dieting. For some, dieting means starving themselves and eating foods that are tasteless. As the text suggests, a person can safely lose weight while still eating reasonable portions of good-tasting food. Remember, a crash diet, losing weight at too fast a pace, is unhealthy. A safe rate of weight loss is 1 to 2 pounds per week. It doesn't sound like much, but it gives the body a better chance to adjust to weight loss and minimizes the risk of medical complications.

If your students want to lose weight, suggest that they try the 1,200-calorie diet recommended in Appendix D (p. 212) of *Y's Way to Water Exercise*. If this doesn't work for them, they may want to try an organized program, such as *Y's Way to Weight Management*.

There are sophisticated methods of monitoring weight loss by keeping exact records of the caloric values of foods eaten and of the amount of calories expended in activity. However, many people don't have the time or patience to use such methods. That's why you as an instructor should stress the basic concepts of weight management. Even when students have reached their desired weight goals, they need to continue monitoring their eating habits and their physical activity patterns. Students can find more detailed information on weight loss in *Y's Way to Water Exercise*, chapter 11, "Weight Conscious: Applying the Magic Formula."

Sharing all this information with your students should help them develop good weight-management practices. They must realize that in addition to applying the basic concepts in this chapter, they need both commitment and discipline to develop good nutrition and weight-management habits. Encourage them to reach these goals.

In the next and final chapter, we will discuss program feedback and how it can help you improve your teaching and your class format.

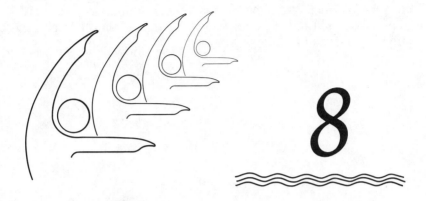

Program Feedback

The success of an exercise program in part depends on its evaluative process. Without feedback from participants about you and the program, you would be denied the opportunity to improve your weak points and build on your strong ones. Allowing participants to evaluate your class gives them the satisfaction that they are able to give input that may improve future classes. Don't worry—not all evaluations are negative. Participants take evaluations seriously and make constructive comments.

Although you may see this as just another administrative task, you'll appreciate both the positive and the negative comments, especially if you have been teaching for some time. After teaching the same activity over and over again, it's sometimes hard to see your teaching objectively. Feedback from the class may reveal some teaching deficiencies that may have developed over time. With some effort you can correct these difficulties.

It is quite possible that your YMCA already has a standard evaluation form that you are required to use. If not, program and instructor feedback forms appear on the next two pages for easy use. You may copy them directly from this manual for distribution to your class. The forms are simple and elicit quick responses, so administering the evaluation should take only a short time.

Y's Way to Water Exercise Instructor Feedback Form

Please rate the instructor on a scale of 1 to 5 (1 = strongly agree; 5 = strongly disagree) on the following items (circle one):

The instructor . . .

1. has a pleasant teaching personality.	1	2	3	4	5
2. is knowledgeable about the subject.	1	2	3	4	5
3. is easily heard when teaching.	1	2	3	4	5
4. is always on time.	1	2	3	4	5
5. is available to discuss my questions.	1	2	3	4	5
6. teaches with the health and well-being of the students in mind.	1	2	3	4	5
7. leads exercises at an intensity level that most of the class can follow.	1	2	3	4	5
8. periodically increases the intensity of exercise during class.	1	2	3	4	5
9. varies the workout enough to make it interesting.	1	2	3	4	5
10. appropriately divides class time among aerobic and upper, middle, and lower body exercises.	1	2	3	4	5
Overall, I am satisfied with the instructor's performance.	1	2	3	4	5

Additional comments:

Y's Way to Water Exercise
Program Feedback Form

Please rate the *Y's Way to Water Exercise* program on a scale of 1 to 5 (1 = strongly agree; 5 = strongly disagree) on the following items (circle one):

The *Y's Way to Water Exercise* program . . .

1. is well organized.	1	2	3	4	5
2. was successful for me, because I made some positive changes in my body.	1	2	3	4	5
3. develops all the components of physical fitness.	1	2	3	4	5
4. should include some swimming activity.	1	2	3	4	5
5. should include more games.	1	2	3	4	5
6. should include a harder workout.	1	2	3	4	5
7. should be offered more often.	1	2	3	4	5
8. was taught in a pool with comfortable water temperature.	1	2	3	4	5
9. used appealing music during exercise.	1	2	3	4	5
10. taught me more about physical fitness.	1	2	3	4	5
Overall, I am satisfied with the *Y's Way to Water Exercise* program.	1	2	3	4	5

Additional comments:

Appendix A

Outline for Minilecture Series

Beginner's Class

Minilecture 1 Orientation to Water Exercise (Class 1)

I. Why people exercise (chapter 4)
   A. To feel good
   B. To look good
   C. To lose weight
   D. For medical reasons
   E. Because society endorses exercise

II. Definition of physical fitness and its components (instructor's guide, chapter 3; participant's text, chapter 1)
   A. Physical fitness
   B. Cardiorespiratory fitness
   C. Body composition
   D. Flexibility
   E. Muscular strength
   F. Muscular endurance

III. Why exercising in the water is beneficial (instructor's guide, chapter 2; participant's text, chapters 1 and 2)
   A. Reduced stress on the body, especially the joints, because a submerged body weighs 90 percent less than one out of water
   B. Effects of resistance
   C. Massage effect
   D. Relaxing environment

IV. The physical properties of water (instructor's guide, chapter 2; participant's text, chapter 2)
   A. Temperature
   B. Resistance
   C. Buoyancy
   D. Massage effect
   E. Pressure

Minilecture 2 Use of Heart Rates in Exercise (Class 2)

I. Training heart rates (instructor's guide, chapters 3 and 4; participant's text, chapter 5)

A. Formula for calculating training heart rate range
B. Necessity of aerobic exercise's lasting 15 to 30 minutes
C. Practice taking pulse counts
D. Effect of drugs on heart rate

Minilecture 3 Facts on Losing Weight (Class 5)

I. Weight loss, diet, and exercise (instructor's guide, chapter 7; participant's text, chapter 11)

A. "Magic formula"
B. Importance of water
C. Safe weight loss of 2 pounds per week
  1. 3,500 calories in 1 pound of fat
  2. Fat burned during aerobic activities
  3. Weight lost according to genetic design or order of gain
  4. Spot reducing: a fallacy
D. Dieting as consuming less food and selecting more nutritional foods
E. Exercising during a diet in order to maintain or increase muscle mass

Minilecture 4 How to Maintain Your Exercise Program (Class 7)

I. Motivational techniques (instructor's guide, chapter 4; participant's text, chapter 17)

A. Peer support
B. Exercising with a friend
C. Establishing a routine
D. Seeing results; compliments

Minilecture 5 Personalizing Your Program (Class 9)

I. How to individualize your workout (participant's text, chapter 5)

A. Identifying personal fitness goals
B. Physical fitness tests
C. Doctor's approval, especially after 35 years of age
D. Standard workout
E. Exercise guidelines and precautions

II. Emphasizing correct form in the exercises (instructor's guide, chapter 4)

A. Avoiding injury
B. Full benefits from exercise

Minilecture 6 Everyone Can Perform Water Exercise (Class 14)

I. Water exercise is for everyone (participant's text, chapters 11 through 15)
   A. The weight-conscious
   B. Pregnant women
   C. People with health problems
   D. People recovering from injuries
   E. Older adults
   F. Athletes

II. Specific health problems and their effects on exercise (participant's text, chapter 13)
   A. Orthopedic problems
   B. Heart problems
   C. Arthritis
   D. Obesity
   E. Lower back problems
   F. Multiple sclerosis

Minilecture 7 Injuries and Water Exercise (Class 17)

I. Reemphasizing proper intensity and progression in the workout (participant's text, chapter 5)

II. Injuries and exercise in the water (participant's text, chapter 14)
   A. Rehabilitative effect on injuries of exercising in the water
   B. YMCA instructors discouraged from prescribing treatments for injuries
   C. Precautions

Minilecture 8 Your Results From Exercise (Class 21)

I. Acknowledging progress individuals make and reviewing benefits of exercise (participant's text, chapters 1 and 5)

II. Preparing participants for posttesting by reviewing test activities

Intermediate Class

Minilecture 1 Motivation (Class 7)

References: instructor's guide, chapter 4; participant's text, chapter 17
  I. Reviewing personal goals
  II. Reasons people drop out of exercise programs
     A. Benefits of exercise not experienced
     B. Injury from muscle overuse or strains
     C. Business schedules taking priority
     D. Exercise program not challenging or interesting
     E. Others
  III. Identifying the motivational technique that works best for each participant

Minilecture 2 Nutrition (Class 14)

References: instructor's guide, chapter 7; participant's text, chapter 11
  I. The expression "you are what you eat"
  II. Roles nutrients play in physical activity
     A. Carbohydrates as the primary source of energy
     B. Fat and proteins as energy-producers after glycogen stores are depleted
     C. Functions of protein, minerals, vitamins, and water in the body
  III. Proper eating habits
     A. Eating a balanced diet
        1. Meats
        2. Dairy products
        3. Fruits and vegetables
        4. Grains
     B. Eight guidelines for eating healthy
  IV. Weight-loss techniques
     A. Dieting without exercise, resulting in loss of muscle mass as well as fat
     B. Importance of exercise
     C. Aerobic activity
     D. Weight-loss goals; 2 pounds per week safe

Minilecture 3 Aging and Exercise (Class 18)

Reference: participant's text, chapter 15

   I. Concerns aging person has about exercise
      A. Health problems that cause restriction of movement
      B. Fear of injury
      C. Embarrassment at awkward movements
  II. Why the older adult should exercise
      A. Exercise important at any age
      B. Physical fitness sets the stage for good health
 III. Why water exercise is particularly good for older adults
      A. Buoyancy of water easier on joints, causes fewer aches and pains
      B. Water massages muscles
      C. Cooling effect of water allows longer, more comfortable workout than on land
      D. Fewer stressors than in other types of exercise
      E. Provides opportunities for socialization

Advanced Class

Minilecture 1 Sports Performance (Class 6)

Reference: participant's text, chapter 16

I. Water exercise's contribution to improving sports performance

    A. Application of the specificity of training principle in the water

    B. Sport-specific water exercises complement an athlete's general conditioning program

II. Examples of sports conditioning programs

    A. Tennis and racquetball

    B. Softball and baseball

    C. Golf

Minilecture 2 Injuries (Class 9)

References: participant's text, chapters 14 and 16

I. Why a person (athlete) may be able to continue to exercise with an injury

    A. Buoyancy allows movement without undue strain

    B. Overload easily controlled

II. Precautions injured person should take when exercising

    A. Must have physician's release to exercise

    B. Watch for symptoms of pain

    C. Exercise in moderation

    D. If prescribed, apply hot and cold treatments

    E. Continue taking prescribed medications

III. Differences between sports injuries and nonathletic injuries

Minilecture 3 Advanced Fitness (Class 11)

References: instructor's guide, chapter 3; participant's text, chapter 16

I. Definition of physical fitness and how it should differ for an athlete or person with advanced fitness

    A. A higher level of physical fitness required

    B. Fitness components developed for specific sport skills

II. How an athlete's conditioning program differs from a nonathletic program

    A. Specific movements practiced to develop nerve or motor pathways for specific skills

    B. Frequency, intensity, and duration increased

Appendix B

Sample 50-Minute Circuit-Training Workout

Procedure

1. Make a sign naming the exercise to be performed at each station. Place these signs strategically around your teaching area for a good student flow pattern.
2. Select a method to signal students to move on to the next exercise, such as blowing a whistle or stopping the music for a few seconds.
3. Divide students into groups. Explain that they should move as a group from one station to another on your signal.

Format

Phase I—Warm-up (3 stations, 2 minutes per exercise)

1. Joggernaut
2. Universal
3. Hip Dip

Phase II—Aerobics (10 stations, 2-1/2 minutes per exercise)

1. Downhiller
2. Cossack Shuffle
3. Heel Slap
4. Side Leg Side
5. Charleston Flap
6. Cheerleader Jump
7. Gerbil Wheel
8. High Jump
9. Joggernaut
10. Jumping Jacks

Phase III—Upper body (3 stations, 1 minute per exercise)

1. Mae West
2. Wing Flap
3. Figure 8

Phase IV—Middle body (5 stations, 1 minute per exercise)

1. Modified Scissors Cross
2. Hula Hoop
3. Body Twist

4. Windshield Wiper
5. Six Count Twister

Phase V—Lower body (3 stations, 1 minute per exercise)
1. Lateral Lift
2. Flamingo
3. Pendulum

The preceding exercises account for 42 minutes. The 8 extra minutes of your 50-minute class session is used up in switching stations and in a 3- to 4-minute cool-down.

Appendix C

Water Games

The following water games can vary the regular water exercise workout. They are divided into those that can supplement the aerobic exercises and those that are just generally fun.

Games With an Aerobic Effect

Relay Races

The class is divided into teams. A starting point and a halfway point are identified. The members of each team line up single file. When the signal to start is given, the lead competitor of each team races to the halfway point, turns around, and races back to the starting line. There he or she tags the teammate next in line, who races back and forth and tags the next teammate. The winning team is the first one whose members all complete the race activity.

Use the following activities for the races:

- Bunny Hop
- Downhiller
- High Jump (leaping forward)
- Chariot Race (walk while towing a person in an inner tube or ring buoy)
- Dead Weight Jog (while walking backwards, towing a person who is vertical but balled up, pulling by the elbows)

The intensity of this game may be increased by requiring each team member to go around the course two or more times before tagging a teammate.

Water Exercise Tag

While every other class member performs the Joggernaut exercise, someone who has been chosen to be "it" jogs around a defined area trying to tag another member. Class members try to avoid being tagged, but must stay within the defined area. This continues for a specified period of time. The winner is the class member who has been tagged the fewest times.

Over and Under

The class is divided into teams of at least four members each. Each team lines up single file. While everyone performs the Joggernaut exercise, the person first in each line passes a ball over his or her head to the person behind. This second person then stops jogging, passes the ball under the legs to the next person, and begins jogging again. This alternating pattern continues until the ball reaches the last person in the line. The ball's direction is then reversed as it is passed back to the first person. The team that first completes passing the ball back and forth through the line is the winner.

Run the Rapids

The class jogs in a circle. At a given signal, everyone turns around and jogs in the opposite direction, against the current (turbulence) created by the circular movement.

Chorus Line Kick

The class forms separate lines of at least four students each. They try to perform the Chorus Line exercise in unison. All the members of each line should connect by interlocking shoulders and arms. Once the lines are synchronized, each line turns clockwise, then counterclockwise, in place.

Inner Tube Water Polo

This is a modified form of water polo. The class is divided into two teams of at least five players apiece. Each team tries to score by putting a ball in the opponent's goal, while defending its own goal. (Goals can be made out of two upright objects about 10 to 12 feel apart.) Each team has a goalie and is divided evenly into offensive and defensive players.

Players are seated in inner tubes and may use their arms and legs to propel themselves. Depending on the distance from the deck to the water surface, the goalie may either sit on the deck in the goal area or sit in an inner tube while defending the goal.

Start the game by having the teams positioned at opposite ends of the pool. Throw the ball into the center of the pool. The ball must be passed among team members at least three times before an attempt to score can be made. All play must be for the ball; no intentional body contact is allowed. The winner is the team with the most goals scored in a set period of time.

Games of Fun

Spin the Wheel

Depending on your class's size, form one large or several small circles (a minimum of six students in each circle), the students facing inward and interlocking their arms and shoulders. Have students in each circle alternately call off as 1s and 2s.

Instruct the 2s to walk sideways, turning the circle, while the 1s do the following movement sequence:

1. Lift legs and lock them in a knees-to-chest position.
2. Extend both legs toward the middle of the circle while the torso is upright, forming a 90-degree angle at the hips.
3. Remain in same position as in step 2 but perform a leg kick.
4. Lie on back (supine) with legs open and extended, touching toes or ankles with other class members in the same position, creating a pinwheel effect.

After the circle has turned twice, 2s should walk while 1s perform the movement sequence.

Water Volleyball

Play modified volleyball if your facility has the equipment. Divide the class into two teams. Position them in waist- to shoulder-depth water. Once the ball is put into play, each team must return the ball over the net to the opposing team within three ball hits. Any part of the hand may be used to hit the ball. Score this game the same as you would a standard volleyball game.

This game could even be played without a net. It's possible to just divide the two teams with a line marker; they then play as usual.

For additional ideas on water games, consult either of these two books.

American Red Cross. (1981). *Swimming and aquatics safety.* Washington, DC: Author.

YMCA of the USA. (1986). *YMCA progressive swimming instructor's guide.* Champaign, IL: Human Kinetics.

Appendix D

Exercises With Water Jugs

Exercises with water jugs can vary the water workout and provide an alternate middle body workout when the regular middle body exercises cannot be used due to lack of a pool gutter. The type of jugs recommended are 1-gallon plastic milk jugs that can be obtained from a local dairy for less than a dollar or brought in by students.

The jugs are used empty and capped when support is needed for a middle body workout. For strength workouts, a gradual increase in resistance can be achieved by starting with jugs half-full of water. Because jugs are less buoyant when filled, moving them through water is easier. In subsequent workouts the jugs can be filled with less and less water, increasing the resistance.

The following exercises work the majority of large muscle groups in the body, especially the stomach, the hips, and the thighs. Each person needs two jugs and should be positioned in water at least shoulder deep. Perform at least 8 to 10 repetitions of each exercise.

Leap Jug

From a standing position with jugs extended horizontally in front of the body, the student jumps forward while sweeping the arms and jugs backward behind the body. The jugs glide along the water's surface. The body ends up leaning slightly forward. The student then jumps backward, with the arms and jugs sweeping to the front of the body. The knees should be lifted high off the pool bottom during the jumping action.

Topsy-Turvy

This exercise uses the same basic movements as the Leap Jug, except the student starts in a floating, face-up (supine) position with arms and jugs extended above the head. He or she starts the exercise by sweeping the arms "down" to the hips while pulling the legs toward the chest and then extending them behind the body. The body ends up in a prone float position. To complete the exercise, this movement is reversed so that the body returns to the supine position.

Six Count Twister

The student performs the regular Six Count Twister exercise, but with the body in a supine position and arms holding jugs extended at 90 degrees on either side of the body.

Floating Jumping Jacks

The student opens and closes the legs using jumping jack movements while floating in a supine position and holding the jugs out to the sides of the body.

Twisted Scissors

From a supine position with arms and jugs extended out to the sides of the body, the exerciser twists the body to the left as far as possible. Once in this position, he or she opens the legs in a scissorlike movement. He or she closes the legs, then repeats the twisting movement of the body to the right and executes the scissor-kick action once again. The exerciser continues these alternating side-to-side twisting and scissor-kicking movements until 8 to 10 repetitions have been performed. The extended arms provide the needed stabilization for the exercise.

Modified Scissors Cross

The regular Modified Scissors Cross can be easily performed with jugs. Instead of holding on to the pool wall, the student extends the arms and jugs horizontally out to the sides of the body. He or she performs the scissors leg motion normally.

Windshield Wiper

The regular Windshield Wiper exercise can also be performed with the arms and jugs in the same position as the Modified Scissors Cross.

Bicycle Pedal

The exerciser starts in a supine position with the arms and jugs extended 45 degrees from the body. He or she performs a pedaling motion with the legs. The stomach muscles can be emphasized by moving the knees as close to the chest as possible. A variation would involve moving the arms in a flutterlike horizontal movement back and forth between the sides of the body and the extended 45 degree position while pedaling.

Appendix E

Health Screening, Medical Clearance, and Informed Consent Forms

The following five forms are taken from *Health Enhancement for America's Work Force—Program Guide* (YMCA of the USA, 1987). They can be reproduced and used as needed for your YMCA classes. The screening forms should be administered when participants enter a program and yearly thereafter. Copies of all completed participant forms should be retained in a records file for at least 3 years.

Form I—Health Screen Form

Form I is the Health Screen Form. It obtains general information about the participant's physical condition. The form is completed by the participant to document information on age, height, weight, blood pressure, smoking, diabetes, heart problems, family history, and orthopedic and other problems. It also includes information on whom to contact in the event of an emergency. Form IA (Range of Recommended Body Weights) is used to determine the classification of current body weight (Question 1). Individuals with heart or other problems that may limit exercise must obtain medical clearance from a physician before being allowed to participate in YMCA fitness testing or exercise programs.

Form II—Cardiovascular Disease Risk Factor Estimate

Form II provides a way to estimate the individual's risk for developing heart disease. It is completed and scored by the participant. (YMCA staff may have to help participants complete the items on blood pressure and heart rate.) Form IA is again used to determine weight category (Question 3). After Y staff have reviewed this form, it is used in an educational process to help participants evaluate some of their health habits and initiate steps to improve their lifestyles. Persons with high-risk scores (33 or greater) are required to obtain medical clearance from a physician before participating in fitness testing or exercise programs.

Form III—Medical Clearance Form

The Medical Clearance Form is used by the participant's physician to report any restrictions that should be placed on the participant during fitness testing or exercise programs. The physician should see both Form III and Form IIIA, which describes generally the YMCA fitness testing and exercise programs and the risks associated with each.

Form IV—Informed Consent for Fitness Testing

The Informed Consent for Fitness Testing form insures that the participant is aware of the risks involved in the fitness testing procedures. It documents that a description of the testing procedures has been read and that all questions concerning those procedures have been answered satisfactorily.

Form V—Informed Consent for Exercise Participation

The Informed Consent for Exercise Participation form insures that the participant is aware of the risks involved in exercise. It documents that the description of the exercise program has been read and all questions concerning the exercise program have been answered to the participant's satisfaction.

When and How to Use These Forms

The Health Screen Form (Form I) and the Cardiovascular Disease Risk Factor Estimate (Form II) should be completed before a participant starts any program, even if it is just an education class. The information obtained in Forms I and II is valuable for determining the level of a participant's health and cardiovascular risk. Note that Forms I and II are not intended to be medical exams but simply to obtain key health information.

Any person who responds affirmatively to Questions 2, 5, 7, or 8 on the Health Screen Form or who scores 33 or higher on the Cardiovascular Disease Risk Factor Estimate may not participate in any fitness test or any exercise program until the Medical Clearance Form (Form III) is completed and signed by a physician.

The informed consent forms (Forms IV and V) are designed to notify participants of the inherent risks of fitness testing and exercise programs. Form IV (Informed Consent for Fitness Testing) should be given to any person registering for a fitness test. It should be read and signed before testing starts. Form V (Informed Consent for Exercise Participation) should be given to any participant in a supervised exercise program. It should be read and signed before exercise starts.

Form I—Health Screen Form

Name _____   Date _____

Male __ Female __ Age ___ Height _____ Weight _____

This form is intended to obtain relevant information about your health that will assist the staff in helping you with your program. Please answer all questions to the best of your knowledge.

1. Weight
   According to the attached recommended weight chart, is your current body weight
   _____ underweight?   _____ 5 to 19 lbs overweight?
   (more than 5 1b
   under ideal)
   _____ normal?   _____ more than 20 lbs overweight?
   (± 5 1b of ideal)

2. Blood Pressure
   Do you have high blood pressure?   yes   no
   Have you had high blood pressure in the past?   yes   no
   Are you on medication for high blood pressure?   yes   no

3. Smoking
   Do you smoke?   yes   no
   Are you a former smoker?   yes   no
   If yes, please give date you quit.
   _____

4. Diabetes
   Do you have diabetes?   yes   no

5. Heart Problems
   Have you ever had a heart attack?   yes   no
   Heart surgery?   yes   no   Angina?   yes   no

6. Family History
   Have any of your blood relatives had heart disease, heart surgery, or angina?   yes   no

7. Orthopedic Problems
   Do you have any serious orthopedic problems that would prevent you from exercising?   yes   no
   If yes, please explain.

   _____

   _____

   _____

8. Other Problems
   Do you have any reason to believe you should not exercise?
      yes   no   If yes, please explain.

   _____

   _____

   _____

9. Emergency
   Please list a relative whom we may contact in case of an emergency:

   Name _____ Telephone _____

   Relation _____

Form IA Range of Recommended Body Weights Health Screen Form

| Height | Weight in pounds | |
	Men	Women
5'0"	—	96-125
5'1"	—	96-128
5'2"	112-141	102-131
5'3"	115-144	105-134
5'4"	118-148	108-138
5'5"	121-152	111-142
5'6"	124-156	114-146
5'7"	128-161	118-150
5'8"	132-166	122-154
5'9"	136-170	126-158
5'10"	140-174	130-163
5'11"	144-179	134-168
6'0"	148-184	138-173
6'1"	152-189	—
6'2"	156-194	—
6'3"	160-199	—
6'4"	164-204	—

Note. From *Implementing Health/Fitness Programs* (p. 111) by R.W. Patton, J.M. Corry, L.R. Gettman, and J.S. Graf, 1986, Champaign, IL: Human Kinetics. Copyright 1986 by R.W. Patton, J.M. Corry, L.R. Gettman, and J.S. Graf. Adapted by permission.

Form II—Cardiovascular Disease Risk Factor Estimate

Name _____

Date _____

1. Age	10-20 Years — 1	21-30 Years — 2	31-40 Years — 3	41-50 years — 4	51-60 years — 6	> 60 years — 8
2. Heredity: parents and siblings	No family history of CVD — 1	One with CVD over 60 years — 2	Two with CVD over 60 years — 3	One death from CVD under 60 years — 4	Two deaths from CVD under 60 years — 6	Three deaths from CVD under 60 years — 7
3. Weight: refer to Form IA	More than 5 lbs. below standard weight — 0	-5 to +5 lbs. of standard weight — 1	5 to 20 lbs overweight — 2	21 to 35 lbs overweight — 3	36-50 lbs overweight — 5	51-65 lbs overweight — 7
4. Tobacco smoking	Nonuser — 0	Occasional cigar or pipe — 1	Cigarettes 10 or less/day — 2	Cigarettes 11-20 per day — 4	Cigarettes 21-30 per day — 6	Cigarettes over 30/day — 10
5. Exercise	Intensive job and recreational exertion — 0	Moderate job and recreational exertion — 1	Sedentary job and intensive recreation — 2	Sedentary job and moderate recreation — 4	Sedentary job and light recreation — 6	Sedentary job. No special exercise — 8
6. Cholesterol and triglycerides	Low-fat diet. No sugar intake — 0	Below-average fat and sugar intake — 2	Normal fat and sugar intake — 3	High-fat and normal sugar intake — 5	High fat and sugar intake — 6	Excessive fat and sugar intake — 8
7. Systolic blood pressure	< 111 mmHg — 0	111-130 mmHg — 1	131-140 mmHg — 2	141-160 mmHg — 3	161-180 mmHg — 5	Above 180 mmHg — 7
8. Diastolic blood pressure	< 80 mmHg — 0	80-85 mmHg — 1	86-90 mmHg — 2	91-95 mmHg — 4	96-100 mmHg — 7	Above 100 mmHg — 9

9. Gender	Female < 40 years (1)	Female 40–50 years (2)	Female > 50 years (4)	Male (5)	Male (paunchy) (6)	Male (obese) (7)
10. Resting heart rate — Men	< 56 (1)	57–64 (2)	65–70 (3)	71–77 (4)	78–81 (5)	> 82 (7)
10. Resting heart rate — Women	< 65 (1)	66–70 (2)	71–75 (3)	76–82 (4)	83–86 (5)	> 87 (7)
11. Stress	No stress (1)	Occasional mild stress (2)	Frequent mild stress (3)	Frequent moderate stress (4)	Frequent high stress (5)	Constant high stress (7)
12. Present CVD symptoms	None (0)	Occasional fast pulse and/or irregular rhythm (2)	Frequent fast pulse and/or irregular rhythm (4)	Occasional angina (6)	Exertional angina (8)	Frequent angina (exertional and resting) (10)
13. Past personal CVD history	Completely benign (0)	CVD symptoms not MD confirmed (2)	CVD mild MD confirmed BP medication (4)	CVD moderate Occasional symptoms (6)	CVD severe frequent symptoms (8)	Hospitalized for CVD (10)
14. Diabetes	No symptoms. Negative family history (0)	Latent positive family history (1)	Elevated blood glucose (3)	Mild dietary control (5)	Moderate oral medication control (7)	Severe insulin control (9)
15. Gout	No symptoms. Negative family history (0)	Family history (1)	Elevated uric acid (> 8 mg/dl) no symptoms (2)	New onset Gout. Medication control (3)	Repeated chronic gouty attacks (5)	Gout with renal and osteo complications (8)

TOTAL SCORE

Remarks: _____

If you score:

6–14 = Risk well below average
15–19 = Risk below average
20–25 = Risk generally average
26–32 = Risk moderate
33–40 = Risk dangerous; you must reduce your score
41–55 = Risk very dangerous; you must reduce your score immediately
56 + = Risk extreme; urgent medical treatment recommended

Note. Adapted by permission of the New York State Education Department's HEALTHY STATE PROGRAM, Albany, N.Y.

Form III—Medical Clearance Form

Dear Doctor:

_____ has applied for enrollment
Name of applicant
in the fitness testing and/or exercise programs at the YMCA. The fitness testing program involves a submaximal test for cardio-respiratory fitness, body composition analysis, flexibility test, and muscular strength and endurance tests. The exercise programs are designed to start easy and become progressively more difficult over a period of time. A more detailed description of the testing and exercise programs is attached in Form IIIA. All fitness tests and exercise programs will be administered by qualified personnel trained in conducting exercise tests and exercise programs.

By completing the form below, however, you are not assuming any responsibility for our administration of the fitness testing and/or exercise programs. If you know of any medical or other reasons why participation in the fitness testing and/or exercise programs by the applicant would be unwise, please indicate so on this form.

If you have any questions about the YMCA fitness testing and/or exercise programs, please call.

Report of Physician

_____ I know of no reason why the applicant may not participate.

_____ I believe the applicant can participate, but I urge caution because

_____

_____

_____ The applicant should not engage in the following activities:

_____

_____

_____ I recommend that the applicant NOT participate.

Physician signature_____Date _____

Address _____ Telephone _____

City and State _____ Zip _____

Form IIIA—Description of Fitness Testing and Exercise Programs

Dear Doctor:

The YMCA fitness testing and/or exercise programs for which the participant has applied are described as follows:

Fitness testing—the purpose of the fitness testing program is to evaluate cardiorespiratory fitness, body composition, flexibility, and muscular strength and endurance. The cardiorespiratory fitness test involves a submaximal test that may include a bench step test, a cycle ergometer test, or a one-mile walk for best time test. Body composition is analyzed by taking several skinfold measures to calculate percentage of body fat. Flexibility is determined by the sit-and-reach test. Muscular strength may be determined by an upper-body bench press test and a lower-body leg extension test. Muscular endurance may be evaluated by the one-minute, bent-knee sit-up test or the endurance bench press test.

Exercise Programs—The purpose of the exercise programs is to develop and maintain cardiorespiratory fitness, body composition, flexibility, and muscular strength and endurance. A specific exercise plan will be given to the participant based on needs and interests and your recommendations. All exercise programs include stretching exercises for warm-up and flexibility development and may involve walking, jogging, swimming, cycling (outdoor and stationary), exercise fitness class, rhythmic aerobic exercise class, choreographed fitness class calisthenics, or strength training. All programs are designed to place a gradually increasing work load on the body in order to improve overall fitness. The rate of progression is regulated by exercise target heart rate and perceived effort of exercise. All programs include warm-up, exercise at target heart rate, and cool-down.

In both the fitness testing and exercise programs, the reaction of the cardiorespiratory system can not be predicted with complete accuracy. There is a risk of certain changes that might occur during or following exercise. These changes might include abnormalities of blood pressure and/or heart rate. YMCA exercise instructors are certified in CPR, and emergency procedures are posted in the exercise facility.

In addition to your medical approval and recommendations, the participant will be asked to sign informed consent forms that explain the risks of fitness testing and exercise participation before the programs are initiated.

Form IV—Informed Consent for Fitness Testing

Name _____

(please print)

The purpose of the fitness testing program is to evaluate cardio-respiratory fitness, body composition, flexibility, and muscular strength and endurance. The cardiorespiratory fitness test involves a submaximal test that may include a bench step test, a cycle ergometer test, or a one-mile walk test. Body composition is analyzed by taking several skinfold measures to calculate percentage of body fat. Flexibility is determined by the sit-and-reach test. Muscular strength may be determined by an upper-body bench press test and a lower-body leg extension test. Muscular endurance may be evaluated by the one-minute, bent-knee sit-up test or the endurance bench press test.

I understand that I am responsible for monitoring my own condition throughout the tests, and should any unusual symptoms occur, I will cease my participation and inform the instructor of the symptoms.

In signing this consent form, I affirm that I have read this form in its entirety and that I understand the description of the tests and their components. I also affirm that my questions regarding the fitness testing program have been answered to my satisfaction.

In the event that a medical clearance must be obtained prior to my participation in the fitness testing program, I agree to consult my physician and obtain written permission from my physician prior to the commencement of any fitness tests.

Also, in consideration for being allowed to participate in the fitness testing program, I agree to assume the risk of such testing, and further agree to hold harmless the YMCA and its staff members conducting such testing from any and all claims, suits, losses, or related causes of action for damages, including, but not limited to, such claims that may result from my injury or death, accidental or otherwise, during, or arising in any way from, the testing program.

_____   _____
(Signature of participant)   (Date)

_____   _____
(Person administering tests)   (Date)

Form V—Informed Consent for Exercise Participation

I desire to engage voluntarily in the YMCA exercise program in order to attempt to improve my physical fitness. I understand that the activities are designed to place a gradually increasing work load on the cardiorespiratory system and to thereby attempt to improve its function. The reaction of the cardiorespiratory system to such activities can't be predicted with complete accuracy. There is a risk of certain changes that might occur during or following the exercise. These changes might include abnormalities of blood pressure or heart rate, ineffective heart function, and possibly heart attack or cardiac arrest.

I understand that the purpose of the exercise program is to develop and maintain cardiorespiratory fitness, body composition, flexibility, and muscular strength and endurance. A specific exercise plan will be given to me, based on my needs and interests and my doctor's recommendations. All exercise programs include warm-up, exercise at target heart rate, and cool-down. The programs may involve walking, jogging, swimming, cycling (outdoor and stationary), exercise fitness class, rhythmic aerobic exercise class, choreographed fitness class, calisthenics, or strength training. All programs are designed to place a gradually increasing work load on the body in order to improve overall fitness. The rate of progression is regulated by exercise target heart rate and perceived effort of exercise.

I understand that I am responsible for monitoring my own condition throughout the exercise program and should any unusual symptoms occur, I will cease my participation and inform the instructor of the symptoms.

In signing this consent form, I affirm that I have read this form in its entirety and that I understand the nature of the exercise program. I also affirm that my questions regarding the exercise program have been answered to my satisfaction.

In the event that a medical clearance must be obtained prior to my participation in the exercise program, I agree to consult my physician and obtain written permission from my physician prior to the commencement of any exercise program.

Also, in consideration for being allowed to participate in the YMCA exercise program, I agree to assume the risk of such exercise, and further agree to hold harmless the YMCA and its staff members conducting the exercise program from any and all claims, suits, losses, or related causes of action for damages, including, but not limited to, such claims that may result from my injury or death, accidental or otherwise, during, or arising in any way from, the exercise program.

_____   _____
(Signature of participant)   (Date)

Please print:

Name _____ Date of birth _____

Address _____
        Street   City   State   Zip

Telephone _____

Name of personal physician _____

Physician's address _____

Physician's phone _____

Limitations and medications _____

Appendix F

Aerobic Exercise Intensity Ratings

The aerobic exercises included in the *Y's Way to Water Exercise* program are rated according to their degree of difficulty or perceived level of intensity. This is based on the premise that some exercises tend to raise the heart rate during exercise significantly higher than others. Previous use of these exercises has also led to this conclusion. The following designations are assigned to each exercise.

1 = high-intensity exercise
2 = medium-intensity exercise
3 = low-intensity exercise

Exercise	Intensity rating	Plane of movement
Bunny Hop	2	Frontal
Charleston	2	Oblique
Charleston Flap	3	Lateral
Cheerleader Jump	1	Lateral
Chorus Line	3	Oblique-lateral
Cossack Shuffle	1	Frontal
Cross-Country Skier	2	Frontal
Downhiller	2	Lateral
Flutter Kick	1	Frontal
Gerbil Wheel	2	Oblique
Heel Slap	3	Oblique
High Jump	2	Frontal
Joggernaut	1	Frontal
Jumping Jacks	3	Lateral
One Leg Hop	3	Frontal
Polaris	2	Frontal
Scissors Jump	1	Lateral
Side Leg Side	2	Lateral

These ratings are based on the exercise being performed at a moderate speed or cadence. It should be noted that it is possible to increase an exercise's rating by increasing the speed at which the exercise is performed. Thus, an exercise rated a 3 may, in effect, become a 2; a 2 may become a 1.

Resources

Books

Cotterman, S.K. (1985). *Y's way to weight management.* Champaign, IL: Human Kinetics.

Golding, L.A., Myers, C.R., & Sinning, W.E. (1982). *The Y's way to physical fitness.* Champaign, IL: Human Kinetics.

Howley, E.T., & Franks, B.D. (1986). *Health/fitness instructor's handbook.* Champaign, IL: Human Kinetics.

Krasevec, J.A., & Grimes, D.C. (1988). *Y's way to water exercise.* Champaign, IL: Human Kinetics.

McArdle, W.D., Katch, F.I., & Katch, V.L. (1986). *Exercise physiology: Energy, nutrition, and human performance* (2nd ed.). Philadelphia: Lea & Febiger.

National Dairy Council. (1983). *Food power: A coach's guide to improving performance.* Rosemont, IL: National Dairy Council.

Wilmoth, S.K. (1988). *Y's way to better aerobics leader's guide.* Champaign, IL: Human Kinetics.

YMCA of the USA and the Arthritis Foundation. (1985). *Arthritis Foundation YMCA aquatic program: Guidelines and Procedures.* Champaign, IL: Human Kinetics.

YMCA of the USA and the Arthritis Foundation. (1985). *Arthritis Foundation YMCA aquatic program instructor's manual.* Champaign, IL: Human Kinetics.

Videotape

YMCA of the USA (Producer), & Witty, C. (Director). (1987). *Y's way to water exercise* [Videotape]. Champaign, IL: Human Kinetics.

Organizations

Aquatic Council
American Alliance for Health, Physical
    Education, Recreation and Dance (AAHPERD)
1900 Association Drive
Reston, VA 22091

National Advisory Committee on Aquatic Exercise
Council for National Cooperation in Aquatics (CNCA)
901 W. New York Street
Indianapolis, IN 46223

President's Council on Physical Fitness and Sports
Judiciary Plaza, Suite 7103
450 Fifth Street, NW
Washington, DC 20001

References

American College of Sports Medicine. (1978). Position statement on the recommended quantity and quality of exercise for developing and maintaining fitness in healthy adults. *Medicine and Science in Sports and Exercise*, **10**, vii-x.

Claremont, A.D., Reddan, W.G., & Smith, E.L. (1981). Metabolic costs and feasibility of water support exercises for the elderly. In F.J. Nagle & H.J. Montoye (Eds.), *Exercise in health and disease* (pp. 215-225). Springfield, IL: C.C. Thomas.

Clarke, H. (1979, February). Definition of physical fitness. *Physical Fitness Newsletter*, p. 1.

Evans, B.W., Cureton, K.J., & Purvis, J.W. (1978). Metabolic and circulatory responses to walking and jogging in water. *Research Quarterly*, **49**, 442-449.

Howley, E.T., & Franks, B.D. (1986). *Health/fitness instructor's handbook*. Champaign, IL: Human Kinetics.

Koszuta, L.E. (1986). Water exercise causes ripples. *The Physician and Sportsmedicine*, **14**(10), 163-167.

Lloyd, A., Thiel, J., Holloman, P., Fletcher, B.J., & Fletcher, G.F. (1986). Water exercise versus land exercise in cardiac patients [Abstract]. *Journal of Cardiopulmonary Rehabilitation*, **6**(10), 434.

McMurray, R.G., Katz, V.L., Berry, M.J., & Cefalo, R.C. (1988). The effect of pregnancy on metabolic responses during rest, immersion, and aerobic exercise in the water. *American Journal of Obstetrics and Gynecology*, **158**(3, Pt. 1), 481-486.

Vickery, S.R., Cureton, K.J., & Langstaff, J.L. (1983). Heart rate and energy expenditure during Aqua Dynamics. *The Physician and Sportsmedicine*, **11**(3), 67-72.

Whitley, J.D., & Schoene, L.L. (1987). Comparison of heart rate responses: Water walking versus treadmill walking. *Physical Therapy*, **67**, 1501-1504.

Additional Resources for Your Aquatics and Health Enhancement Programs

See the YMCA Program Store Catalog for details about these additional items or contact the Program Store, Box 5077, Champaign, IL 61825-5077, (217) 351-5077.

4915	Y's Way to Water Exercise (208 pp)	$9.95
4928	Y's Way to Water Exercise Videotape (VHS, 28 minutes)	$29.95
4740	Y Skippers Manual (240 pp)	$20.00
4912	Parents' Guide to Y Skippers (64 pp) (individual)	$4.00
4938	Parents' Guide to Y Skippers (set)	10/$32.00
4732	YMCA Progressive Swimming Program Instructor's Guide (112 pages)	$10.50

Available Spring 1989:

5003	The Polliwog Swim Book (24 pp)	
5004	The Guppy Swim Book (24 pp)	
5005	The Minnow Swim Book (24 pp)	
4880	Aquatics For Special Populations (168 pp)	$15.00
4957	YMCA Aquatics Program and Leadership Training (40 pp)	$5.00
4720	Arthritis Foundation YMCA Aquatic Program Instructors' Manual (46 pp)	$5.50
4719	Arthritis Foundation YMCA Aquatic Program Guidelines and Procedures (58 pp)	$6.50
4456	Swimming Fitness Card	50/$3.50
4276	Swimming Fitness Award Certificate	50/$5.25
4277	Swimming Fitness Progress Folder	50/$5.25
4271	Swimming Fitness Emblem	10/$9.00
4272	5 Mile Chevron	10/$6.00
4273	10 Mile Chevron	10/$6.00
4274	20 Mile Chevron	10/$6.00
4275	50 Mile Chevron	10/$6.00
4483	100 Mile Chevron	10/$6.00
4484	200 Mile Chevron	10/$6.00
4506	500 Mile Chevron	10/$6.00
552	For Fun and Fitness Mileage Progress Chart	$1.75

Price shown are subject to change.